S
Bone

MW01104965

"*Everyone needs to read this book so we can end osteoporosis.*"   **Mark Victor Hansen**, Coauthor of Chicken Soup for the Soul

"*I love your book. It will be a great benefit to patients at our center and in every doctor's office.*"
John Rumberger, PhD, MD, FACC

"*Dr. Shaffer has essentially constructed a 'How To' primer for women of all ages. Using clear and concise language and gentle explanations, this work guides women through the process of making sensible and sensitive choices for the benefit of their own personal health. I would love to see "Secrets" on the recommended reading list for every teenage girl and expectant mother, and on the personal booklist of every woman who dares to live lifelong in a state of wellness.*"   **Janice Katz Gargan, M.D**.

"*Wow! That document is very impressive. I like it for a lot of reasons: personal story to get involved made me want to read it. Broken up into sections of a length that informs and also maintains interest. Very holistic, educational, motivates and encourages a change in lifestyle from many aspects. I covers a **ton of information** that is **easily digestible for a layman**. You have done a **fabulous job** in organizing and delivering scientific and lifestyle information. Kudos!!*"
Diane Gross, Naturopathic Midwifery Program Coordinator, Bastyr University.

"*Who would have dreamt that osteoporosis would make such a **riveting read**! You have rendered the material masterfully, with insights, personal experience, hard-core data, and best of all, what to do now.*"   **Cheryl, MEd, MS**

"*I read the whole thing, learned a lot! I **was really impressed** with the information and the way it was presented...never gets boring.*"   **Gwyneth SW, Grandmother in PA**

"*The Guide is very **impressive**: Thank you for this great information!*"   **Dave Bailly, Tax Attorney & Accountant**

"*This book is **the best gift you could give** to yourself and anyone you care about. You'll get **new research** on smart nutrition, effective exercise and stress mastery. You can be part of ending osteoporosis by using and sharing the information in this book.*"   **Robert G. Allen, Author of Nothing Down.**

"*...very timely and important health issue...fantastic read...a must for anyone...well researched and engagingly presented.*" **Roxane Polak, PhD, Psychologist**

Secrets Inside
Bones, Brains & Beauty™

Erla, you've enriched my life for decades... THANKS! Build Better Bones, Joyce

Secrets Inside

Bones, Brains & Beauty

Joyce Shaffer, PhD

Osteoporosis Updates
Bones, Brains & Beauty™, LLC
Bellevue WA 98009

© 2005 Joyce Shaffer
ISBN 0-9770411-0-7

All rights reserved. Printed in the United States of America.
No part of this publication may be produced, stored in a
retrieval system or transmitted in any form or by any
means, electronic, mechanical, photocopying, recording or
otherwise without the written permission of the publisher.

Notice to Readers: Information provided here is for
educational purposes only and is not a substitute for
medical advice. This information is designed to support,
not replace, the relationship that exists between a
patient/site visitor and his/her existing physician. If possible,
I will answer your factual questions. Sometimes I will
suggest that you ask your physician for a referral to a
specialist, but I will not give any medical advice. If errors
are brought to our attention, we will try to correct them. Our
goal is to keep this information as timely and accurate as
possible.

Publisher: Osteoporosis Updates
PO Box 765
Bellevue WA 98009-0765

Cover design by Cynthia Pena
Cover pictures by Dr. Joyce

Acknowledgements

The most stellar among us throughout the course of history have accomplished their great deeds with the help of a team. The more we learn from them and follow their model the greater our own success. This writing preserves that model that served them so well...thank you, All.

That team begins with Robert Allen and Mark Victor Hansen. Being in your Inner Circle is to be gifted beyond measure! This book is only one of the contributions the enlightened minds of your Inner Circle will bring to the world with your tutelage. Mentoring comes in shades of grace. Joycebelle, you are the master mentor! Thank you for getting me started correctly. Rita Losee, Jeanette Monosoff and Ruth King – each of you had special expertise to bring.

Theresa Luquette...your business expertise, wise counsel, supportive listening, brilliant perspective and ability to redirect some of my activities in balanced and productive channels has been valuable beyond my wildest imagination. Donna Fox and Paulie Sabol, you have helped me launch this valuable text as well as related efforts in preventing and treating osteoporosis. I also appreciate Jim Scott for putting wind beneath my wings.

For changing the longer words of dedicated science into something closer to poetry, for adding beauty and interest through visuals, and for turning some raw data into an invitation to see the ultimate model of hope, I thank my editor, Stacey Iglesias. Without the help and challenge of my dear friend, Mark Sumpter, I never would have found her. Nor would I have found Cynthia Pena whose design added lightness and grace most fitting for the ultimate model of hope.

Without the support, encouragement, corrective feedback, love and caring of my friends and family, this never could have been written. First and foremost in this group is my miracle mate, Rich. Jay, thanks for your patience, understanding and encouragement. Again.

Protégé friends, Odyssey 2000 bikers, and many others have helped me immeasurably. Allison Brucker, you made my software sing. Diane Gross, your belief in me makes my wheels spin faster. For helping reduce the first rough draft to better reading I thank Diane Cook, Eileen Marra, Kathryn Tracy, Michael & Lynnette Lindemood, Colleen Stutzman, Marian Dull, Gwyn Whitfield, Lori & Chuck Jackson and others too numerous to mention. What a gift to have such wonderful members of my team dedicated to sharing the Ultimate Model of Hope for improving health. To the rest of you who know you've helped I thank you from the depth of my heart and bones.

I wish the ultimate in health, hope and vigorous longevity to each of you and to every reader. It is a privilege to share all that I learn.

Namaste,

Dr. Joyce

Joyce Shaffer, PhD
Empowerment Expert

Bones, Brains & Beauty™, LLC

vi

Table of Contents

Section Two: Calcium and Your Bones

Section Three: Beyond Calcium – Focus on Nutrition, Protein, and Vitamins

Section Four: Exercise to Build Better Bones

Closing Summary and Prediction

References

x

*I'd never seen Grandma
cry before!*

*She'd been my safe
haven…my best model of
strength…more sure than
the Rock of Gibraltar!*

*Now this little old lady
with the hint of a widow's
hump just mumbled
through her tears about
how it held her back –
that cast protecting her
broken wrist.*

*Broken pulling
weeds…just as she had
done all her many years.*
                Gene

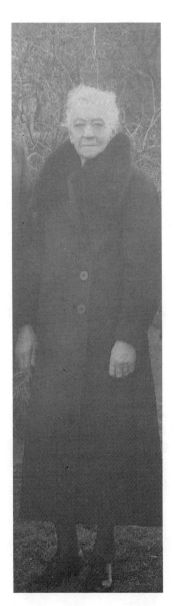

Section One: Understanding Bone Health

A personal experience with bone health

I finally made the decision in early 2002. I'd had reservations about hormone replacement therapy (HRT) for years, but then I would make the routine office visit to my gynecologist (for whom I continue to have tremendous respect) and he would put my mind at ease. This gentle, compassionate, physician always had a firm grasp of the facts of current research. He also offered a clear, learned interpretation of those facts. His overview, arguments, and conclusions had always been clear and convincing. Staying on HRT seemed wise in the face of all that was known.

However, my intuition in early 2002 was to stop taking estrogen and progesterone. I wanted to get a measure of my bone mineral density BMD before doing so, just to establish my baseline. The research indicated that BMD could be negatively affected by discontinuing estrogen replacement therapy. I wanted to be able to compare my current BMD with my BMD after stopping the estrogen to be sure I wasn't doing myself harm. I assumed my current baseline reading would be very good.

Was I ever wrong! My baseline BMD indicated that I had osteopenia. As will be apparent in the definitions that follow, osteopenia is the stage between normal BMD and osteoporosis.

That news was totally discombobulating! I was born on a farm. I milked those cows. I drank that milk then and continued to do so in measured amounts across my entire life.

Not only that, I also think of myself as physically fit. After all, I am one of 250 bicyclists who cycled in and out of 45 countries during the year 2000 averaging 80 miles per day with the Odyssey 2000™ bicycle trek. Click on "bicycling" at **http://www.BonesBrainsAndBeauty.com** for a free copy of the article on that trek. Getting ready for that ride required a lot of training on my bicycle for the 5 years prior to departure!

Also, throughout my entire career in universities and major medical settings I've stayed as well informed as time allowed – just as most other healthcare providers do. I thought I was managing my diet, supplements, and exercise for maximum health benefits. What could I possibly have missed? What was I doing or NOT doing so that I was totally surprised to be diagnosed with osteopenia?

That's what started this whole research project you are reading. Self-preservation!

From reading previous studies, I had learned that osteoporosis is preventable and reversible. Apparently there was additional information that I needed to know about in order to make my own healthcare more effective and protective. I continue to be determined to make osteopenia a temporary visitor even though I did choose to discontinue HRT.

I dove into the research. One of the first surprises was that bicycling is not included in the recommended exercises. At first I thought, "They are obviously studying the wrong bicyclists! Since muscle action and weight bearing are both important to building strong bones, the studies couldn't have limited their research to those bicyclists who stand up when they pedal."

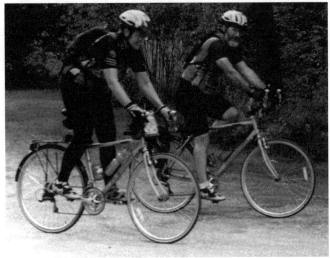

Photo by Kathryn Tracy

And then I remembered – I almost never stood up when I pedaled. Prior to reading this research I sat while pedaling!

Of greatest value to most readers will be the biggest surprise of all: there are so many factors that can influence our bone health, strength, flexibility, and resistance to fractures. That gives us the ultimate model of hope because most of these factors fall into the category of lifestyle choices. Even where we lack any choice, such as in which genes we will inherit, lifestyle choices can modulate the effect our genes will have on our bones.

The more I learned, the more I realized that sharing this knowledge was an obligation. Apparently, so did the US government.

3

The Surgeon General's Report

The Surgeon General has released the "first-ever" report on our nation's bone health. Bone Health and Osteoporosis, A Report of the Surgeon General, was announced in a news release 14 October 2004. You can obtain your copy at **http://www.surgeongeneral.gov**. Follow the links on that site through Reports and Publications. The good news is that many stellar scientists, physicians, and public health experts contributed to this report.

Though the work of these fine scientists is admirable, it is a fact that it can be incredibly difficult for so many minds to agree on any subject. Therefore, the report is very conservative in its recommendations and often doesn't reflect the true findings of many competent researchers at the head of their field. The other thing to remember is that, by the time written reports become available, new research has often been published.

Thus, the inspiration for this guide as well as my website and the email newsletter you can get at **http://ww.BonesBrainsAndBeauty.com**. In these electronic formats it will be possible to keep the public up to date on the late breaking news regarding research on bone health. After you have finished reading this guide, I invite you to visit the website regularly to keep abreast of new findings on osteoporosis and bone health. Research is constantly evolving and I am committed to keeping my readers well informed.

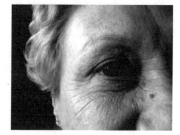

What to expect from this guide

In the following pages you'll learn ways to determine if you might be at risk for low bone density. Even if you discover that your bones aren't enjoying optimal health, remember; it's never too late to start building strong bones.

We'll explore what researchers say may reduce your bone loss and strengthen your bone tissue. Through good nutrition, exercise, the use of the proper supplements, becoming an expert in your own stress management and other sound lifestyle choices, you'll be able to improve your bone health regardless of your age.

Osteoporosis and Osteopenia Overview

What Is Osteoporosis?

Osteoporosis – and **osteopenia** – are defined by bone mineral density (BMD) as compared to the peak bone density of a healthy young adult. The definition is based on how many standard deviations (SD) your score is above or below the mean, or average, for a healthy young adult.

Population	Bone Mineral Density (BMD)
Normal	1 SD above or below the mean
Osteopenia	-1 to -2.5 SD below the mean
Osteoporosis	-2.5 or more SD below the mean
Severe Osteoporosis	>-2.5 SD below the mean AND there has been one or more fracture without severe trauma. A "Widow's Hump" is the hallmark symptom.

Risk factors for Osteoporosis and Bone Fracture

- **Low bone mineral density (BMD)**

- **Being 75 years old or older whether male or female;**

- **The risk is higher among women who**
  - Are **Caucasian or Asian** in ethnicity
  - Have always been **thin**;
  - Were **tall at the age of 25**;
  - Were **never pregnant**;
  - Rated their **health** as **fair or poor**;
  - Had chronic **inflammation;**
  - Had **bone turnover indicated in urine tests**;
  - Had previous **hyperthyroidism**;
  - Had been **treated with long-acting benzodiazepines or anticonvulsant drugs**;
  - **Ingested greater amounts of caffeine;**
  - Were **smokers**;
  - Were **heavy alcohol users**;
  - Did not **exercise regularly**;
  - **Spent four hours a day or less on their feet.**

- **Functional factors associated with increased risk of fracture include**
    - The **inability to rise from a chair without using one's arms**;
    - **Right and left foot coordination**;
    - **Poor depth perception**;
    - **Poor contrast sensitivity**, AND
    - **Tachycardia** (fast heart rate) at rest;

- **Fracture risk is also increased with the risk of falling as predicted by**:
    - Being **thin and frail**.
    - **Slower gait speed**;
    - **Difficulty in doing tandem (heel-to-toe) walking**;
    - **Reduced visual acuity**;
    - **Small calf circumference**; AND
    - **Impaired physical strength and balance.**

Important Facts to Remember:

1. **Women do not have a monopoly** on OSTEOPOROSIS – osteoporosis in men is less frequent but can be more deadly.

2. **OSTEOPOROSIS is a silent disease.** Too many of us are suffering from poor bone health, but we may not realize the fact before it is too late.

3. Even young **fitness buffs can suffer overuse injury** when they over-train to the extent that demineralization of their bones occurs.

4. **OSTEOPOROSIS is** underrated, poorly investigated, and **not treated adequately in a large number of people who are at risk.**

5. **Global increases in "Third Age" people** (men & women 60-plus years old) **will cause a dramatic increase in osteoporotic fractures.**

6. OSTEOPOROSIS is **NOT part of normal aging. It can be prevented and treated!**

7. Most importantly; **It is never too late to build better bones.**

Even with a family history of osteoporosis, LIFESTYLE CHOICES made by you CAN IMPROVE YOUR BONE HEALTH & DECREASE YOUR RISK OF BONE FRACTURES. This reading tells what you can do, at any age, to decrease the effects of this debilitating disease.

Understanding Bone Structure

In order to fully understand the effects of osteoporosis, we must first explore tho unique roles played by our bones. Though some people assume that bones are fixed and rigid, bone is an extremely active organ within our bodies. Our bones are constantly at work.

Bone mass is composed of special proteins called collagens as well as cells and minerals. Continual remodeling of bone takes place through life as well as when micro-damage occurs. Remodeling is done by two types of cells. **Osteoclasts** remove small amounts of bone. **Osteoblasts** are then recruited to the excavation site to create new bone.

Bone differs from all other body tissues in two very important ways. First, 70 to 90% of bone is *inorganic* minerals. These minerals include primarily calcium and phosphorus which are critical to harden the bone. Second, a uniquely large proportion of a bone's total *organic* material is collagen. The proteins making up this collagen are critical in setting the size, shape, and structure of your bones. The organic part of a bone is 90% collagen as compared to most soft tissues, like skin and muscle, which contain 10% collagen.

What is true for any structure is also true for bones. There are three things that influence strength:

Density

The first of these is the density of the materials the object is made of. For example, a given length of bamboo has less density or mass than the same measure of steel. Bone mineral density, or bone mass, is critical to bone

9

strength. Generally, the higher your bone mineral density, the stronger your bones are. In this way our skeleton is comparable to other structures.

Physical Qualities

The second factor influencing strength is any unique physical qualities of the materials used in building the object. To use the same example, bamboo is more flexible than steel. A balance of the right nutrition and mechanical stress influences which kinds of materials will be in your bones.

When you get enough protein, energy and other important nutrients, the basic structure of your bones can store more calcium and phosphorus to harden the bones. With a healthy balance of good nutrition and adequate physical activity, you build the materials into your bones that can handle stress without the ultimate failure, i.e., fracture.

Spatial Relationships

The third thing that determines strength is how these materials are put together in space. Whether made of bamboo or steel, the structure will be more stable if pieces are put together to form a triangle than it would be using the same material to make a square. When the mechanical stress is gradually increased and your bones are remodeled, the proper nutrition supplies what is needed to put your bones together for increasing maximum strength.

Why Modern Medicine focuses on Density

There are several reasons that modern medicine has focused on bone mineral density (BMD) when assessing the strength of the human skeleton. Bone density can be measured in living human beings without surgery or other invasive methods. Also, measuring the two other factors of strength in living human bones has not been possible.

Measuring density is a reliable way to measure strength, however. Mathematically, the strength of a structure is approximately equal to the square of tho density of that structure. Therefore the measure of density will lead us to a measurement of overall strength.

Another reason for focusing on bone mineral density is that we can exercise some control over it. Because our bones are constantly rebuilding themselves, if we take the proper steps to modify our behavior with regards to nutrition and exercise, we can actually increase our bone density and improve the strength of our skeleton.

This is why our bones are able to deal with "fatigue". You may have seen how a piece of metal will break if it is bent back and forth frequently enough. It is the "fatigue" that the metal undergoes from the frequent bending that accounts for metal breaking.

It's to our advantage that our bones repair the damage of fatigue. This is one of many ways that they are unique among structures. They repair and remodel damaged areas. This remodeling process can even strengthen the existing structure to accommodate heavier loads than were carried on our bones before the damage occurred.

Bone density is also important when concerned with the likelihood of bone fracture. BMD is strongly predictive of risk for fractures at all ages. The lower your BMD, the higher your chance of sustaining a break. Increasing BMD in youth is especially effective for reducing the risk of fracture in the present as well as on a long-term basis.

How is bone mineral density measured?

Bone mineral density is measured by a DXA scan. That stands for dual energy X-ray absorptiometry. You may see this abbreviated as "DEXA" or "DXA" scan. Most commonly this scan will focus on measuring one or two particular areas.

The DXA scan measures the bone mineral density or mass in the areas of interest. Absolute accuracy is not possible with this test because it does not fully correct for body size. That means it does not account for small stature. It does not even account for changes during growth. Even so, there are more reasons to use this measure of BMD than there are arguments against it.

It is recommended that both the spine and the hip be scanned to increase accuracy of the assessment of risk for any kind of fracture. The hip and spine are the two sites that most frequently fracture. If only one site is chosen to be measured, then a measurement of the hip is considered preferable to a measurement of the spine. In part, that is related to the more serious consequences from a broken hip than from a fracture of a vertebra in your spine.

That being said, it is also significant that all cases of osteoporosis do not have the same underlying cause. It is illogical to treat every case in the same way. Even with a genetic predisposition to osteoporosis, other measures besides the DXA bone scan may be part of your healthcare provider's assessment.

Urine and blood tests might be included in your assessment. It would be important to find out whether osteoporosis is in an active phase, such as during post-menopausal periods, or whether the bone mineral density is stable even if it is low. Also, it might be appropriate to measure how well your body is absorbing calcium.

See Appendix C for some of the additional tests your healthcare provider might recommend. However, it will be the DXA scan that will be used to come to a diagnosis of osteoporosis or osteopenia.

The Importance of Peak Bone Mass

Peak bone mass is achieved in the hips prior to age 20 years. For most of the rest of the body peak bone mass is accomplished by the age of 30 years. However, the femur (hip bone) and vertebral bodies (of your spine) continue to increase in diameter.

This usually also includes increases in stiffness of the bones and in their capacity to carry weight. In other words, this usually increases bone strength. Interestingly, the skull also increases in bone mass throughout life.

Bone health at any point in time is a reflection of what has happened across your entire life. That includes the time prior to birth. All things considered, bone mineral density is similar across your life. In other words, a person who is at the high end of BMD compared to the rest of the population at age 25 will probably be at the high end at age 85.

Some researchers suggest that a tendency to develop osteoporosis could be identified even before adolescence. In any case, the higher your peak bone mass is in early life, the better chance you have of avoiding fractures later in life, all things being equal.

What do genes have to do with it?

About 75% of the influence on peak bone mass is set by genetic factors according to some scientists. This statement is based on research with twins and non-twin siblings. Some of the genetic influence is related to hormones.

Human growth hormone is one example. In healthy 24-year-old men, about one-third of the difference in bone mass was related to differences in peak nighttime growth hormone secretion. Since lifestyle factors such as exercise also influence the secretion of growth hormone, the amount of genetic influence cannot be clearly determined.

How your body handles vitamin D, sex hormones and insulin-like growth factor (IGF) is also influenced by your genes. Even with these, it is very difficult to calculate the amount of impact that comes from what you inherit in your genes versus what you influenced by your lifestyle choices.

On the one hand, it is clear from twin studies that genetic factors are important in determining BMD. It is also clear that several genes have an impact. By the same token, it is virtually impossible to separate genetic from environmental influence. Even with a genetic predisposition for problems, environmental changes can compensate.

For example, assume a person is genetically predisposed for inefficient absorption and use of nutrients. If they have a higher intake of these nutrients through their diet or supplementation, their BMD will be similar to someone who is more efficient in absorption and use of nutrients. It is important to remember that most of the genetic factors are subject to the influence of environmental factors. That's why personal empowerment is your ultimate model of hope.

For these reasons, a family history of osteoporosis should only be used to encourage you to make the lifestyle choices that will allow you to achieve maximum peak bone mass. In other words, just because your mother had osteoporosis, don't assume that you will have it as well. **BMD is not ruled by genes alone. You can make behavioral changes that will protect your bones.**

In a study of daughters of mothers who had osteoporosis, measures of bone health were more similar in the mothers than in the daughters. The difference in the daughters whose bone health was best could be explained by differences in their nutrition, exercise and other lifestyle choices.

Adolescence: The Window of Opportunity

Adolescence is a brief window of opportunity. It is the age when you can have maximum effect on building your peak bone mass. It is the period when it is the most important to protect and enhance this bone building process.

If an unfortunate circumstance derails bone building, it would be essential to make every effort to compensate for these interruptions. Examples of events that could decrease the rate at which you build your bones include:

- **A long period of bed rest or immobilization;**

- **Inadequate food intake, particularly of calcium, protein or vitamin D;**

- **The onset of eating disorders;**

- **The development of severe generalized illness; or**

- **The interruption of production of normal reproductive hormones such as the loss of menstrual periods once they have started.**

These problems at any age leave the individual at risk for bone loss. During adolescence they take a worse toll than at any other age. This increases the likelihood of entering adulthood at the low end of bone mineral density. A low BMD during younger years predicts that you will continue to have a low BMD during later years. What this

16

means is that you will then be at a higher long-term risk for having a fracture.

Depositing calcium in our bones is like putting money in the bank – too few people do enough of either. Evidence keeps coming in that life-long calcium intake improves bone mineral density and decreases risk of fractures. During adolescence is when we can create the greatest benefit with adequate deposits. That's sort of like accumulating compound interest on your money in savings.

Unfortunately, during adolescence more than half of the boys are consuming less than 77% of the recommended amount. Even so, they do better than the girls. Nearly 90% of adolescent females are consuming less than 77% of the recommended intake of calcium.

Perhaps it's time to help adolescents find independence, identity, peer approval, physical beauty, and other healthy outcomes in different choices. What if we could show them lifestyle choices that are fun, easy, and bound to build better bones? Research shows that this is do-able!

Learning to make constructive, healthy choices is a skill that would serve them well across their entire life. There are so many ways to help prevent – and even reverse – osteoporosis! In fact, it's never too early and never too late to deposit bone strength for health, safety and vigorous longevity.

Nutrition and Bone Mass

The cells of your bones require total nutrition just like any other cell in the body even though their function is different. These bone cells deposit, maintain, and repair your bones and require a wide variety of fuel in order to work properly. In later sections we'll explore ways to use a

Secrets Inside **Bones, Brains & Beauty**

healthy diet and supplementation to supply the body with the necessary nutrients for optimal bone health. The following will explain to you how these nutrients are used in the creation of bone structure.

How Nutrients Influence Bone Mass

Bone cells are responsible for building the matrix which forms the basic and most flexible part of the structure of your bone. Making this matrix requires the production and modification of a special kind of protein called collagen. Your bone cells also produce a variety of other special proteins. All of these types of protein are essential in bone health.

To accomplish these responsibilities the cells of your bones need adequate protein, energy, vitamins and minerals just to build this matrix. This matrix gives shape and structure for your bones. It also holds the mineral deposits that harden your bones while increasing your BMD.

The bony matrix also serves as a warehouse for calcium and phosphorus. The amount of the calcium and phosphorus in bony storage depends in part on the daily balance between how much you swallow and absorb of these two elements and how much of each one is excreted.

Since calcium is the nutrient most likely to be consumed in amounts far below current recommendations, it gets the most attention in research. That's why your healthcare provider is likely to recommend that you count your calcium. This is also why we'll be concentrating solely on Calcium in our next section.

18

Hormones and Bone Mass

Bone loss is accelerated when women's production of the hormone estrogen drops dramatically after menopause. This happens to a lesser degree as men decrease testosterone production with age.

Benefits of Hormone Replacement Therapy (which helps to replace lost estrogen) in post menopausal women include a 34% decrease in risk of osteoporotic hip fractures. DHEA in men was shown to increase spinal BMD, while use of the parathyroid hormone is an encouraging new treatment.

Phytoestrogens (plant based sources of estrogen), called isoflavones, can preserve BMD. One study says that isoflavones from clover and soy consumed orally and in amounts less than 2 mg per kilogram of body weight should be considered safe. A kilogram is about 2.2 pounds. So this researcher is suggesting that a daily intake of less than 1 mg of soy isoflavones per pound of your body weight can be considered safe.

Post menopausal women with habitually high intakes of dietary isoflavone were found to have higher Bone Mineral Density values at both the spine and hip region. Eating even 10 grams (typical Asian intake) of isoflavone-rich soy protein per day may be associated with health benefits. This would be only about 15% of the total USA protein intake.

Special Considerations for Bone Health

Pregnancy and Breastfeeding

Research shows many changes during both of pregnancy and breastfeeding can affect bone mass. However, these effects seem to be temporary. Apparently they do not increase the risk for osteoporosis. Later measures of bone density are not decreased. The risk for fracture in not increased.

A recent study looked at a group of women who had six or more pregnancies and breastfed them for at least six months. In essence, they were either pregnant or breastfeeding most of their adult life. Their bone mineral density was as healthy as the comparison group of women who had never been pregnant.

Apparently the rapid changes of hormones with so many pregnancies and periods of breastfeeding did not interfere with bone health. It is worth considering whether the extra physical activity that is likely to be part of caring for so many children had some impact on these findings. More research is needed on this topic.

There are many benefits to breastfeeding including a lower risk of breast cancer and cancer of the reproductive organs. Modifying nutrition and physical activity to accommodate the demands of breastfeeding can be as simple as following your healthcare provider's advice.

Smoking, Alcohol & Caffeine

These are threats to bone health that you can control. Don't smoke. It reduces bone mineral density and leaves you at greater risk for fractures. Even without smoking, you may be at risk for these bad effects if you are exposed to household tobacco smoke. It is the nicotine and the cadmium in the smoke that is harmful to your bone cells. Women who were exposed to tobacco smoke in their homes during adolescence had lower bone density in adulthood. So just don't smoke. And don't hang out near somebody else who does.

Drinking alcohol may cause you to lose more calcium and magnesium from your body. It also might reduce the rebuilding of bone because of the way it affects the behavior of Vitamin D in the body. In addition, alcohol damages the bone cells that build new bone. Alcohol increases your risk for fracture, possibly by increasing your risk for falling. Excessive alcohol use usually also results in poor nutrition and liver disease.

Caffeine intake was studied in a group of women who were healthy and between the ages of 66 and 77. At the beginning of the study the bone density of the two groups was similar at all of the bone sites measured. Three years later bone loss at the spine was significantly higher in the group that had consumed more than 300 mg of caffeine per day.

The hip and total body measures of bone density showed more bone loss with the higher caffeine intake after 3 years. Caffeine was also found to alter a genetic predisposition for bone remodeling. Therefore, greater than 300 mg of caffeine per day may reduce your bone density. 18 ounces, about 3-4 cups, of regular brewed coffee would probably be the equivalent of 300 mg.

The impact of stress

We've learned a lot from different forms of culture. In this example I'm referring to the cultures used in research laboratories to study the impact of environmental influences. Admittedly, part of my fascination with this particular study comes from the way it ties in with my expertise in stress management. Let's return to that after learning more about this research on bone cells in culture.

The bone volume is reduced with osteoporosis and osteopenia. Along with that the fat tissue in your bone marrow is increased. Scientists hope that being able to reverse that might be a novel therapy to treat osteopenia and osteoporosis.

They have learned that there are certain human bone cells that get to make a career choice. If these bone cells are placed in a culture with 1,25-dihydroxyvitamin D3 (a form of vitamin D), they become osteoblasts. Put more simply, the bone cells given appropriate vitamin D matured into the type of bone cells that Build Better Bones.

However, another selection of similar bone cells was given a very different culture. They were placed in chemicals similar to those your body produces under mental or physiological stress. This is to be distinguished from the mechanical stress you put on your bones when you jump – which leads to building strength in your bone. Bone cells influenced by the chemicals of stress matured into adipocytes, otherwise know as fat cells.

Granted the story of this research is much more complex than the scope of this writing allows. But the goal of these researchers is a worthy one: To reduce the number of cells that mature into fat cells and increase the number of bone cells that mature into bone-building osteoblasts.

The logic of this would suggest that mastering stress management might be another lifestyle choice to help you Build Better Bones. The smorgasbord of choices you have to master stress adds to the Ultimate Model of Hope.

Stress is.

There are skills to help you reduce the occurrence of trauma. There are additional tools to reduce the ravages of stress on your body during unfortunate situations.

One of the greatest gifts you can give yourself is learning how to go from misery to mellow in seconds. For more information go to **http://www.StressPower.com**.

Fractures

There are two times across the lifeline when fractures are most frequent. Although the most research has been done with women during and after menopause, the first increase in frequency of fractures occurs during puberty at about the time of the growth spurt. For girls this is between the ages of 11.5 and 12.5 years. For boys, this is between 13.5 and 14.5 years of age. At this age about two thirds of the fractures are caused by light trauma.

Typically, **light trauma** refers to falling to the floor while standing on the floor or sitting on furniture. In contrast, falling off a step-ladder would not be light trauma.

The wrist is the most common site. It accounts for almost a fourth of all fractures during growth. According to research, one third of all fractures in children could not be related to a specific activity or environment. Many wrist fractures in adolescents fit the criteria of *fragile* bone fractures and might be compared to those called "osteoporotic" in adults.

Stress fractures are overuse injuries. They are a result of accumulation of stress from repetitive loads that are lower than would be required to fracture bone in a single-injury situation.

When a bone is subjected to a new level of stress, it is normal for the bone to remodel its structure and density to increase its strength. That includes removing any evidence of wear and tear followed by adding new bone that is better able to bear the heavier load. There are special bone cells that work together to accomplish this miracle of healing.

Usually the removal of the stressed part of the bone does not weaken the bone sufficiently to be a problem in the short run. Normally the new bone is added rapidly enough to correct any weaknesses or to repair any micro-damage.

However, when the wear and tear is repeated faster than the bone can be fully repaired, the bone is more fragile than usual. Complete failure at this point would be a fracture due to stress which ordinarily would not have caused a fracture. These are seen most frequently in young athletes or dance enthusiasts in serious training.

Low BMD increases the risk for stress fractures because less dense bones bend to a greater degree than massive bones do. Because of that they get more damage from fatigue. To decrease your risk of stress fractures, it is recommended that you increase your level of activity gradually and avoid sustained, excessive activity.

Hip and spine are also common sites affected. Fractures of the vertebrae can occur without any symptoms.

The possible implications of a fracture

In a study published in June 2004, the occurrence of fracture did not increase the likelihood of drug treatment for osteoporosis. The implication of this, of course, is that

24

both clinicians and their patients are not as knowledgeable about the possible implications of a fracture as they need to be.

Any fracture that results from a light trauma fall can reasonably be considered a risk for osteoporosis. Remember, a light trauma fall includes falling to the floor from standing upright or from sitting in a chair. Therefore, if you experience such a fracture, it makes sense that you would be tested for osteoporosis and possibly treated with the appropriate lifestyle changes and, perhaps, medications.

Inflammation, immunity and osteoporosis

It's important to understand the role of inflammation in the "thinning" of bones. Inflammation is a part of your immune response that reacts to any encroachment, damage or trauma to your body. Examples include when you cut your finger, get food stuck between your teeth, get dust in your eyes or fracture a bone.

Your brain sees this problem, sends out an SOS and dozens of tiny chemical are released to the site of the problem. Each chemical is part of helping you overcome the problem. The bad news is that some of these chemicals which are released as a mechanism of protection can actually become harmful. Too much of a good thing is not always helpful.

In the case of your bone mineral density, some of these chemicals prevent the thickening and layering of calcium onto bone thus preventing bone healing. By focusing on the chemicals which control inflammation, researchers have begun to understand the inflammatory process and to discover countermeasures.

It is equally important to understand how your lifestyle choices interact with the inflammatory process. Cholesterol, for example, has been shown to promote the inflammatory processes. Stress, particularly depression, has an adverse effect on regulating the inflammatory process. This is the Ultimate Model of Hope again because diet and stress mastery as under your voluntary control.

A patient's responsibility

It can seem easy to blame doctors for a lack of attention to bone health. Remember: Nobody can read the entire library. No doctor, no matter how diligent, has the time or energy to read every medical research report or to keep themselves entirely up to date on the latest medical developments on every important topic.

Besides, you are the only one in the world who will ever spend 24 hours a day with you. No one else can ever be as accurate as you are in measuring and modifying your own lifestyle choices. The gift of personal empowerment is what sets you free to build optimal bone health.

Therefore, if you are risk-averse in any realm of your life, let that be the case in terms of your bone health. Learn everything you can about how to Build Better Bones. Discover the latest medical advances and research findings. Also be aware of the way in which cultural and gender bias may affect your medical treatment. Then ask your health care provider questions as an informed consumer – as the person with the most investment in your own health status.

You may be more vulnerable because of family history or lifestyle choices. If you have any reason to suspect that you are at increased risk for osteoporosis or any disease, make it your obligation to make your doctor aware of this increased risk.

For example, many more women than men reported discussing osteoporosis with their doctors. This is probably largely due to the fact that osteoporosis is still culturally considered to be "a women's disease." Those women who had these discussions were consistently advised to increase their calcium and vitamin D intakes.

The amount of calcium supplements did increase significantly in these women. However, an increase was not found in men. Therefore, more women than men received consultation as well as calcium and vitamin D supplements as treatment for osteoporosis.

Again, your role as a consumer gives you the firmest grounds for hope. The more informed you are, the better your questions are when you begin the conversations with your healthcare provider about treatment options. You are empowered by being your own best advocate.

Putting your bone knowledge to use

Once you understand the function of the skeletal system and the factors that influence bone health, you're ready to start putting that knowledge to use. In the following sections we'll explore the important roles that calcium, proper nutrition and supplementation, stress management and exercise play in building the strongest bones possible.

Secrets Inside Bones, Brains & Beauty

Section Two: Calcium and Your Bones

Good reasons to double your calcium intake immediately.

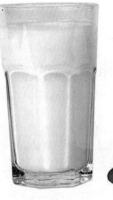

Almost 100 percent of the US population is consuming *half* the amount of calcium that is recommended as the minimum daily requirement. However, almost everyone believes they are getting enough of this essential mineral. For that reason, we need to focus on calcium before we explore other necessary vitamins and minerals.

The glass of milk pictured here with the gingersnaps is one example of how to get calcium in what you drink and eat. The milk would supply about 300 mg of calcium. Depending on what recipe was used to create the gingersnaps, 23 or more mg of calcium would be found in each cookie. You can get extensive information at **http://www.nal.usda.gov/fnic/foodcomp/Data/SR17/wtr ank/wt_rank.html**. That government source of data on nutrients in your food is very valuable. Some examples follow.

> ### *Calcium*.
> Recommended daily intake of calcium are within the following ranges:
>
> | | |
> |---|---|
> | **0-6 Months** | **210 mg** |
> | **7-12 Months** | **270 mg** |
> | **1-3 Years** | **500 mg** |
> | **Preadolescent children** | **800 to 1200 mg** |
> | **Adolescents & young adults** | **1200 to 1500 mg** |
> | **Adults** | **1000 mg** |
> | **Men & women ages 50 or older** | **1000 to 1500 mg** |

What choices do we have?

Eat Smart

Build to your strengths by eating smart. The Framingham Osteoporosis Study found that a **high fruit and vegetable intake** appeared to be protective in men. Diets high in candy were the most unhealthy for bones in both sexes. It seems that carbohydrates that come naturally packaged in fiber are critical to our health - especially when very little processing has been done to them before we eat them.

Malnutrition has also been associated with osteoporosis. Certain basic needs must be met. These include minerals, vitamins, hormones, fats, carbohydrates and proteins. Information offered in this report on Recommended Daily Allowances (RDA) were adapted from the Dietary Reference Intakes (DRI) reports. For more

Secrets Inside Bones, Brains & Beauty

information on the Dietary Reference Intakes, see
http://www.nap.edu.

In many nations the main sources of dietary calcium are milk products and green, leafy vegetables. The value of milk products as a source of calcium for some people is evident. Both Croatia and China give us good examples.

In Croatia, District A consumed more dairy products than was natural to District B. District A had about twice as much calcium intake as District B. Hip fractures were less frequent in the elderly of District A than in District B.

In China, women aged 35 to 75 years living in five rural counties were investigated. These women in pastoral counties had higher dairy calcium and total calcium intake than the women living in non-pastoral counties. Women with the higher dairy sources of dietary calcium increased bone mineral density by facilitating optimal peak bone mass earlier in life.

We know that other things also influence our bone mineral density, but inadequate calcium intake in the foods we eat is one of the most important. Doctors and nutritionists recommend getting about 500 mg of calcium at every meal since the body can only properly absorb a fairly small amount of calcium at a time. It's worth repeating that almost no one gets an adequate intake of this all-important mineral.

This doesn't have to be the case. The choices of foods that are calcium rich are a gourmet's delight. Even the non-gourmet has plenty of options. Whether you're making a calzone packed with calcium rich ricotta cheese and broccoli, or simply packing raisins in a sack lunch, you can make choices that will introduce more calcium into your diet.

Secrets Inside Bones, Brains & Beauty

The United States Department of Agriculture is a great source for discovering more about the nutritional benefits of the food we eat. Their website gives us some guidance on foods that are rich in calcium. Some of that information is grouped here, divided into food categories.

Dairy Products

What You Eat	What Calcium You Get	
Ricotta Cheese, part skim milk	1 cup	669 mg
Swiss Cheese	1 ounce	224 mg
Provolone Cheese	1 ounce	214 mg
Mozzarella Cheese	1 ounce	207 mg
Cheddar Cheese	1 ounce	204 mg
Muenster Cheese	1 ounce	203 mg
Milk shake, thick vanilla	11 fl ounces	457 mg
Milk shake, thick chocolate	10.6 fl ounces	396 mg
Plain yogurt, skim milk, 13 grams protein	8 ounces	452 mg
Plain yogurt, skim milk, 12 grams protein	8 ounces	415 mg
Eggnog	1 cup	330 mg
Milk, nonfat	1 cup	306 mg
Milk, 1% milk fat	1 cup	290 mg
Milk, chocolate, low fat	1 cup	288 mg
Buttermilk, cultured, low fat	1 cup	284 mg
Milk, nonfat, instant dry	1/3rd cup	283 mg
Ice milk, vanilla, soft serve cone	1 cone	153 mg
Cottage cheese, 1% milk fat	1 cup	138 mg
Cottage cheese, creamed	1 cup	126 mg
Ice Creams, French vanilla, soft serve	½ cup	113 mg
Ice Creams, vanilla, light	½ cup	106 mg
Frozen yogurts, chocolate, soft serve	½ cup	106 mg
Frozen yogurts, vanilla, soft serve	½ cup	103 mg

Secrets Inside Bones, Brains & Beauty
Cereals & Grains

General Mills TOTAL Cereal	¾ cup	1104 mg
Corn meal, self rising, degermed,		
Enriched, yellow	1 cup	483 mg
Cornbread made with 2% milk	1 piece	162 mg
Bread crumbs, dry, grated, seasoned	1 cup	218 mg

Fruits & Vegetables

Papaya	1 papaya	73 mg
Raisins, seedless	1 cup	73 mg
Orange	1 cup	72 mg
Blackberries, raw	1 cup	42 mg
Collards, frozen, chopped, cooked, boiled,		
drained, without salt	1 cup	357 mg
Soybeans, green, cooked, boiled,		
drained, without salt	1 cup	261 mg
Turnip greens, frozen, cooked,		
boiled	1 cup	249 mg
Kale, frozen, cooked, boiled,		
drained, without salt	1 cup	179 mg
Okra, frozen, cooked, boiled,		
drained, without salt	1 cup	177 mg
Beet greens, cooked, boiled,		
drained, without salt	1 cup	164 mg
Chinese cabbage, cooked, boiled,		
drained, without salt	1 cup	158 mg
Broccoli, raw	1 cup	41 mg.

Fast Foods

Taco	1 large	339 mg
Taco	1 small	221 mg
Tostada with guacamole	1 tostada	211 mg

Secrets Inside Bones, Brains & Beauty
Fish

Atlantic sardine canned in oil,
 drained, with bone   3 ounces   325 mg
Salmon, pink, canned, solids
 with bone and liquid   3 ounces   181 mg
Atlantic ocean perch, cooked
 dry heat   3 ounces   116 mg

Soy

Tofu, firm, prepared with calcium sulfate
 and magnesium chloride (nigari)
                      1/4th block   163 mg
Tofu, soft, prepared with calcium sulfate
 and magnesium chloride (nigari)
                      1 piece   133 mg

Miscellaneous

Blackstrap molasses   1 Tablespoon   172 mg
Pumpkin pie   1 piece   146 mg

These options are just the beginning. As you'll soon read, the potential recipe combinations are to live for. Incidentally, if dairy products aren't a fit for you, try adding some of the other items on the list to your food. A little tofu in your fruit smoothie or raisins sprinkled on a salad can add interest as well as calcium to some of your favorite recipes.

Other tips for increasing calcium are substituting canned salmon with bones for tuna fish in making sandwiches, salads, fillings, or on a bagel. Chop tofu or tempeh into salads or stir fry dishes. Use broccoli, kale, okra, turnip greens, collards, and beet greens regularly in

Secrets Inside Bones, Brains & Beauty

soups, salads, or other recipes. Add blackstrap molasses or powdered milk to recipes. Mixing nonfat yogurt instead of sour cream or mayonnaise in recipes is another option. For even more inspiration, consult Appendix E.

Also, many foods are now fortified with calcium. Read labels to check for this. One example is the addition of calcium citrate malate to some brands of orange juice.

Recipes for Increasing Calcium
A RECIPE A DAY (COULD KEEP A FRACTURE AWAY?)

Crisp Corn Griddle Cakes
About 10 thin 2-inch cakes

If you make this version with more liquid, the cakes become lacy and crisp. They're pretty, crunchy, and delicious (according to readers)! Bring olive oil in your skillet to the proper temperature while mixing the ingredients. One test of the temperature is that a drop of water bounces off the heated oil. We use olive oil for its nutritional values. Incidentally, we prefer to limit the fat content of this recipe to the amount absorbed in frying the griddle cakes. Also, some people will prefer to sift the dry ingredients. However, we are "quick gourmets" who require easy and limited effort that can be accomplished in about 10 minutes or less. We just put, stir, and fry ASAP.

Place in a bowl:
$2/3^{rd}$ cups yellow corn meal (about 322 mg calcium)
½ teaspoon salt
$1/4^{th}$ teaspoon baking soda
$1/8^{th}$ cup whole grain flour

Stir these together *briefly*. Then add:
        1 to 1 $1/4^{th}$ cup low fat buttermilk (284 to 355 mg calcium)

Stir the liquid into the dry ingredients with a few swift strokes. Fry immediately. Make the cakes small for easy turning.

Calcium content per whole recipe will be approximately 606 to 677 mg. That makes it a great breakfast source of calcium for two people.

REMEMBER: You want to take in no more than 500 mg of calcium per serving to get the most absorption for each delicious mouthful.

Winter Whole Wheat Pasta

12 ounces of whole wheat spaghetti pasta (138 mg calcium)

Boil pasta according to directions. Cook until al dente. Drain and cover.

In a large skillet, mix together the following. Add carrots, garlic and onions first. After 8 to 10 minutes, add the rest of the ingredients and cook for 5 more minutes.

1 Tablespoon olive oil
1/3 cup red wine
1 Tablespoon minced garlic (15 mg calcium)
2 cups finely chopped Swiss chard (36 mg calcium)
2 1/2 diced onions (88 mg calcium)
1 cup diced carrots (42 mg calcium)
3/4 cup diced celery (30 mg calcium)
1 1/2 teaspoon salt
Ground pepper to taste

Mix sauce (211 mg calcium) with pasta (138 mg calcium) and toss. Top with grated Romano cheese (302 mg per ounce) to taste. 16-ounce serving has approximately 10 grams of fiber.

Asian Vegetable Soup

5 cups vegetable broth
2 cups diced onions (70 mg calcium)
1 1/2 cups diced firm tofu (made with calcium sulfate) (759 mg   calcium)
1 1/2 cup peeled and chopped carrots (53 mg calcium)
1 1/2 cups chopped baby bok choy
1 cup mushrooms, either straw (18 mg calcium) or shitake (4 mg   calcium)
3 minced garlic gloves (15 mg calcium)
1/2 cup cilantro (6 mg calcium)
3 tablespoons soy sauce
1 1/2 tablespoons fresh grated ginger
Minced scallions for garnish

Place broth, onions, garlic and carrots in a large soup pot. Simmer for 10 to 15 minutes until desired tenderness. Add all other ingredients (921 mg calcium) and let simmer just until all vegetables are hot. (Remember, overcooking vegetables will begin to leach them of their nutritional value.)

Healthy Hash browns

The hash browns:
8 cups potatoes shredded with skin (160 mg calcium)
2 large garlic cloves, minced (10 mg calcium)
2 cups sliced or shredded onions (70 mg calcium)
3 tablespoons olive oil or no fat olive oil spray
Salt and pepper to taste

Heat olive oil in a large skillet. Sauté onions and garlic until the onions begin to turn translucent. Add the potatoes and lower the heat slightly. Cook 5-10 minutes with the skillet covered, stirring occasionally. Uncover the skillet and cook for 10 more minutes, stirring occasionally.

Secrets Inside Bones, Brains & Beauty
The healthy part:
5 cups of sliced Swiss chard (90 mg calcium), spinach (150 mg calcium), or other 'dark leafy green'
1 1/2 cups green pepper (23 mg calcium)
1 1/2 cups red pepper (15 mg calcium)
1 teaspoon sage (12 mg calcium)

Add above ingredients (200 mg calcium) to the skillet of potatoes (240 mg calcium), reduce heat and cover. Cook a few minutes until greens and peppers are just becoming tender.

Cantaloupe Delight

1 cup nonfat milk (306 mg calcium)
2 ½ cups diced cantaloupe (35 mg calcium)
1 teaspoon stevia fiber

Place all ingredients (341 mg calcium) in blender and process until smooth and frothy. Drink immediately. Makes 2 servings at about 150 mg calcium.

Chocolate Banana Heaven

1 cup nonfat milk (306 mg calcium)
2 large, ripe bananas (14 mg calcium)
1 Tablespoon cocoa (7 mg calcium)
1 Tablespoon stevia fiber

Place all ingredients (327 mg calcium) in blender and process until smooth and frothy. Drink immediately.

Taking Calcium Supplements as indicated

The Harvard review of a large body of research objectively demonstrates the value of adding nutritional supplements to your daily regimen. They can aid in the prevention and/or treatment of diseases or specific risk factors for diseases, including osteoporosis. The American Medical Association has recommended nutritional supplements subsequent to that review.

No matter how nutritious your diet, chances are you won't be able to get an adequate supply of calcium simply through the food you eat alone. There are a wide variety of factors that contribute to dietary deficiency of calcium.

Some people find it difficult to get adequate calcium because of lactose intolerance or a busy schedule with little time to devote to preparing proper foods. Too many others have opted to drink things other than milk – such as cola drinks or other beverages that have no calcium as well as high amounts of sugar.

Even those people who strive to prepare healthy meals rich in calcium, however, may still have difficulty achieving proper levels of calcium and other nutrients. We live in a world where genetically engineered food and pollution can compromise the nutritional value of the food that we eat. Therefore, supplementation can be a good choice for helping our bodies to have adequate supplies of calcium.

Consult your doctor for calcium supplement recommendations and empower yourself by doing your own research as well. The more you educate yourself prior to the office visit, the better your questions will be. Being an informed consumer is more critical today than it ever has been. The health of your bones may be one of your best educational investments. Since more than one form of calcium supplement is available, you will want to learn about several of them.

One of the most important requirements for a calcium supplement is that it must be easily absorbed by the body. Before it can be absorbed, it has to be dissolved. To test your calcium supplement, put it in a small glass of warm water or vinegar. If it has not dissolved within 30 minutes, it probably will not dissolve in your stomach either. You might want to look for another source of calcium.

Calcium Citrate Malate

- Has approximately 40% more absorption than other forms of calcium.

- Reduced bone loss in the spine of postmenopausal women by 60% compared to placebo and compared to calcium carbonate.

- Increased bone mineral density in the hip and wrist of men and women 65 years old and older.

- Reduced fractures when taken with Vitamin D.

- Increased bone mineral density when taken with protein supplements.

Also, read the label to determine the actual amount of calcium in the supplement. This is usually referred to as elemental calcium. This will determine how many tablets you need to take to get enough calcium.

The absorption rate of calcium carbonate, calcium citrate, calcium lactate and calcium gluconate are similar to the rate that calcium is absorbed from milk products. **Calcium Citrate Malate** has shown approximately 40% more absorption than calcium carbonate.

For example, a supplement of 300 mg of calcium in the form of Calcium Citrate Malate would yield absorption of 105 to 126 mg of calcium delivered into your blood stream as compared to approximately 75 to 90 mg that actually makes it into your system from milk or many of the more common calcium supplements such as calcium carbonate or calcium gluconate.

Calcium citrate malate in late postmenopausal women reduced bone loss in the spine by 60% in comparison to placebo and calcium carbonate. Bone mineral density actually increased at the hip and wrist with calcium citrate malate in these women.

A later study looked at men and women who were 65 years of age or older and living in their community. The treated group added 500 mg of calcium citrate malate plus 700 IU of vitamin D3 (cholecalciferol) per day for three years. This combination moderately reduced bone loss in the hip, spine, and total body in these men and women.

Since this improvement was still evident after three years, this suggests long-term effectiveness of supplementation in terms of the skeleton as a whole. Also, a reduced incidence of nonvertebral (non-spine) fractures was noted.

Another study found reduced risk of fractures in elderly women treated with 1200 mg of calcium plus 800 IU of vitamin D. This reduction in fractures was not found when vitamin D was given without calcium. Vitamin D is essential for proper calcium absorption and will be discussed more later in this section.

What else is important about the calcium you take?

You should space your calcium intake out across the day. For one thing, by consuming part of your calcium at bedtime and another part first thing in the morning, you can compensate for the bone loss that can occur during sleep at night. Also, your body can only absorb a certain amount of calcium at one time.

Just as with food, you should take no more than 500 mg of your calcium supplement at any one time. That will maximize the amount that your body will absorb. With certain supplements, eating a meal just before you take your calcium can also be beneficial. Many supplements will break down more quickly with the presence of stomach acids that increase during times when food is introduced to the body.

Calcium citrate malate avoids the problem of having to take your calcium supplement at mealtime, however. That's because it does not require the stomach acid to dissolve the molecules so they can be absorbed.

Calcium and Prescription Medication for Osteoporosis

High calcium intake is especially important when taking prescription medications for osteoporosis. It is calcium and phosphorus that harden the bone structure. Regardless of the medication, all work best with adequate calcium intake.

For example, bisphosphonates (brand names such as Fosamax or Actonel) have been approved by the FDA for use in both prevention and treatment of osteoporosis. They decrease the action of the osteoclasts, the bone cells that are responsible for breaking down bone. This drug family is more effective when combined with calcium supplement treatments.

Though side effects are relatively uncommon with these medications, some patients have reported abdominal and musculoskeletal pain after taking the medications. Others cite increased instance of heartburn and irritation of the esophagus. Appendix C provides more information on the various medication options available.

Why all the fuss about calcium?

Fracture protection

This may be the most critical reason for doing everything possible to keep your bones healthy. Adding 500 mg per day of calcium citrate malate plus 700 IU vitamin D yielded a 54 to 64% reduction in fractures in humans 65 or older living freely in their community. Once again we see the importance of calcium, especially when combined with the proper dose of vitamin D.

The Secret Life of Bones

Nearly everyone is consuming **half** the amount of calcium that is recommended as the minimum daily requirement. Most people do not realize that they are not getting enough calcium. The secret life of bones includes drastic decline in bone health with no symptoms. Waiting until you have a fracture to find out about your bone health is like waiting until you have a heart attack before checking your cholesterol. Too many people do both. Count your calcium…you probably need to double your intake of it.

The Importance of Vitamin D

Vitamin D serves your health in several ways. Each of these affects your bone health and your safety.

For starters, vitamin D is required to form the helper protein that carries calcium across the wall of your intestines into your blood stream. Without this the calcium you've swallowed just passes on by and is flushed down the toilet. With adequate vitamin D you have a better chance of getting the most out of the calcium you swallow. Studies that increased calcium intake without adequate vitamin D showed less improvement in bone density than when vitamin D was added along with the calcium.

Additionally, the reduced risk of fractures found with vitamin D supplements might be related to the ability of vitamin D to decrease the risk of falls. The activity of vitamin D in the muscles could explain this. It may be responsible for helping your muscles be stronger so that you are more stable. Since falls account for most of the fractures in osteoporosis, this role of vitamin D is critical in your overall bone health.

Depression is another risk factor for falls. A fascinating study compared the effects of vitamin D at an adequate intake of 600 IU per day versus 4000 IU per day. IU has been used to indicate the number of International Units of vitamin D. To put that in the language of the newer Dietary Reference Intakes (DRIs), no RDA has been established. However, the "Adequate Intake" (AI) of vitamin D is expressed as micrograms. 1 microgram of cholecalciferol is equal to 40 IU of vitamin D. The adequate intake starts at 5 micrograms (200 IU) for people from birth through age 50 years including pregnancy and lactation. It advances to a high of 15 micrograms (600 IU) for women older than 70 years.

So, the fascinating depression study gave either 15 micrograms or 100 micrograms of vitamin D to patients. Both doses improved their wellbeing. Patients taking the higher amount of vitamin D, however, improved more on this measure of wellbeing. Since depression increases the risk of falling, vitamin D may be reducing fall risk by lessening depression as well as strengthening muscles.

With regard to bone density, the addition of 700 IU of vitamin D supplementation along with calcium citrate malate up to a daily intake of 1300 mg calcium resulted in a significant gain of about 1% in bone density in the spine. This combination of supplements also reduced fractures by 50% in healthy men and women aged 65 or older.

Sunlight supplies most of our vitamin D requirement. Even elderly individuals with adequate sun exposure can achieve increased blood concentrations of vitamin D. Good food sources include cod liver oil and oily fish such as salmon, mackerel and sardines. Eating oily fish 3 to 4 times a week will help satisfy the requirement for adequate intake.

Some recent research findings will help you and your healthcare provider determine your personal optimal intake of vitamin D. Former indications that **5 micrograms (200 IU)** to **15 micrograms (600 IU)** per day would be adequate deserve a closer look.

Recent research suggests these amounts are inadequate. A consensus evolved among experts who analyzed the data. They found that **700 to 800 IU per day appear to reduce fracture risk. 800 to 1000 IU of cholecalciferol per day for adults may be necessary.**

To get a picture of how much vitamin D that really is, there are about 100 IU of vitamin D in a glass of milk or fortified orange juice and about 360 IU in a 3 ounce serving of salmon. Supplements containing vitamin D3, cholecalciferol, could be a realistic way to increase your intake.

So, how will the adequate intake of vitamin D for you be determined? A team of scientists say that you need to keep your blood level of 25(OH)D, one form of vitamin D, above 72 nanomols per liter to prevent osteoporosis. Your healthcare provider can help you determine what your blood level of this form of vitamin D is and how much you may need to consume to keep it above this level. This is one of your baseline measures that will assure that your efforts are tailored specifically to your body's unique needs.

Other Important Minerals

RESEARCH FINDINGS

Other Minerals your bones need each day:

Phosphorus	**1,741 (Plus or Minus 535) mg**
Sodium	**2,400 mg or less per day**
Copper	**900 micrograms**
Zinc	**8 mg for females & 11 mg for males**
Manganese	**1.8 mg for females & 2.3 mg for males**
Magnesium	**320 mg for women & 400-420 mg for men** (Magnesium should be ½ of the amount of calcium)
Boron	**No more than 20 mg**

Magnesium

We need about half as much magnesium as calcium for our bodies to process the calcium. Both minerals along with phosphorus contribute to increasing

Secrets Inside Bones, Brains & Beauty

bone mineral density. In the Framingham Osteoporosis Study magnesium intake was associated with better hip bone density in both men and women. The quality of bone structure is improved by magnesium. Females, particularly teenagers, may be more at risk for inadequate intake of this mineral.

The **RDA of magnesium for adult women is 320 mg** a day and for **men is 400-420 mg** a day. Selected food sources of magnesium include green leafy vegetables, unpolished grains, nuts, meat, starches, and milk.

Phosphorus

This mineral is as important as calcium in making your bones hard. It is needed in every cell of your body. About 85% of the phosphorus in your body is in your bones. It is less of a focus for concern because it is so available in foods commonly eaten.

1741 ± 535 mg each day was beneficial for maintaining bone mineral density in adult men when calcium intake was adequate (1200 ± 515 mg). The **RDA ranges from 700 a day for adults to 1250 mg a day during adolescence.** These numbers do not change during pregnancy and lactation. Dietary sources include milk, yoghurt, ice cream, cheese, peas, meat, eggs, some cereals, and breads.

Copper

Copper is also not a large focus of concern because we tend to get enough in our diets. However, it does play a critical role in making the proper structure of the collagen in our bones. It is part of the enzyme that helps knit the strands of collagen together for the best mechanical strength. For **copper** the daily **RDA is 700 micrograms for pre-adolescents, 890 micrograms for** adolescents, 900 micrograms for adults, 1000 micrograms during pregnancy and 1300 micrograms during lactation. For adults the Upper Limit is 10,000 micrograms per day. Dietary sources include seafood, nuts, seeds, wheat bran cereals, whole grain products, and cocoa products.

Zinc

Zinc also has a role in several enzymes. Some of these influence how various minerals make your bones hard. Others are essential in how your collagen forms the structure of your bones. It is an important part of how our body uses protein. The daily **RDA of zinc for adults is 8 mg for females** and **11 mg a day for males.** For pregnant females this increases to 13 mg during adolescence and 11 mg for adults. During lactation this increases to 14 mg during adolescence and 12 mg for adults. The Upper Limit for daily intake of zinc is 40 mg. Dietary sources include fortified cereals, red meats, and certain seafood.

Manganese

Manganese is another element that helps enzymes work properly to form the protein framework of your bones. It helps regulate the protein for stronger bones. **Manganese has a daily Adequate Intake of 1.8 mg for women and 2.3 mg a day for men. This increases to 2.0 mg during pregnancy and 2.6 mg during lactation.** The Upper Limit is 11 mg per day. Dietary sources are nuts, legumes, tea, and whole grains.

Sodium

Sodium intake should be carefully monitored. 1.5 grams per day is considered an Adequate Intake. However, the average person in the USA swallows a great deal more than that. This is, in part, due to the increasing reliance on fast foods.

Keep this in mind. The sodium and calcium that gets into your blood stream follow similar paths through your kidneys. This is part of the reason that your sodium intake influences how much calcium you lose. For each 57 mg of sodium you eat you lose about 1 mg of calcium in your urine. The American Heart Association set an upper limit of recommended sodium intake for adults at 2,400 mg per day. *Count yours*. That may help you get the most value out of the calcium you swallow.

Boron

Calcium absorption may be improved by boron. Boron might also increase the effect of estrogen. **Boron has no RDA** but its daily Adequate Intake is 11mg during preadolescence, 17 mg during adolescence and 20 mg throughout adulthood. These numbers do not shift with pregnancy and lactation. The **Upper Limit** for adults is **20 mg** a day. Selected food sources include fruit-based beverages and products, potatoes, legumes, milk, avocado, peanut butter, and peanuts.

Fluoride

New bone formation might be stimulated by fluoride. This may explain why habitual tea drinking of more than 10 years had a good effect on bone density of the total body, spine and hip in adults. Teas are a source of fluoride. Adequate Intake is 10 mg daily from preadolescence throughout life.

5 Easy Steps to Build Better Bones

What is our ultimate model of hope with so many nutrients to be considered?

The benefits of studying the many nutrients required to Build Better Bones are huge! The more you know about them, the more you can decide what to measure. The more you learn about your current state of bone health, the better equipped you are to improve it. You can become the choreographer in this intricate dance of the many nutrients required for your bone health. What that means to you is that you have a lot of complex but easy and fun ways to influence your bone health by taking 5 Easy Steps that spell **B O N E S**.

- Step 1 **B** BASELINE measures: Count your intake of these nutrients…because you probably need to increase some of them.

- Step 2 **O** ORGANIZE your own unique winners strategy…so you CAN Build Better Bones. Your options are many and varied. Make them address your baseline measures so those measures can improve.

- Step 3 **N** Now! Do it NOW! Do it with relish…so you can find new and different ways to eat for fun and bone health, too.

- Step 4 **E** Evaluate AND REINFORCE! Give yourself a lot of positive reinforcement for progress…so you can stay on track. Once again, take heart…**osteoporosis is NOT part of normal aging.**

- Step 5 **S** START again from Step 1…so measures of changes in your bone health just keeps getting better and better guided by new science.

Remember...

It is never too early

And never too late

To

Build Better Bones.

Secrets Inside **Bones, Brains & Beauty**

Section Three: Beyond Calcium – Focus on Nutrition, Protein, and Vitamins

Nutrition for Bone Health – Have you counted your total nutrition today?

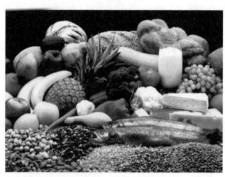

We learned in our last section how important a wide variety of minerals are to our total bone health. In order to achieve an adequate daily intake of these minerals and other important nutrients, you need to focus on eating a complete diet. This isn't a book on proper nutrition, but what you eat has a tremendous effect on your overall bone health. Therefore, a quick overview of what would constitute a healthy diet is definitely worth our time.

A helpful aid is the Food Guide Pyramid. With the incredible amount of diet and nutrition information available today, it's hard to believe that the good old-fashioned food pyramid would retain any relevance, but it remains a useful tool for creating a healthier and more complete diet.

At **http://www.mypyramid.gov/** you can personalize your Food Guide Pyramid for optimal health.

The United States Department of Agriculture created the food pyramid to help people understand the different varieties and quantities of food they should try to include from each food group in their daily diet. By choosing wisely from these groups, we can boost our intake of calcium and of all the other nutrients that can influence our overall bone health. There are a lot of delicious food choices which will help us Build Better Bones at any age with stress mastery and physical activity.

Serving Recommendations from the Food Guide Pyramid Might Be:

Grains	6 ounces, at least half Whole Grain
Vegetables	2 ½ cups, eating a variety
Fruits	1 ½ cups
Milk	3 cups non fat
Meat & Beans	5 ounces
Oils	Aim for 5 teaspoons of oils a day
Discretionary Calories	Limit extra fats & sugars to 195 calories

One size doesn't fit all. Go to **http://www.mypyramid.gov** to get YOUR personal guidelines from the USDA.

Grains

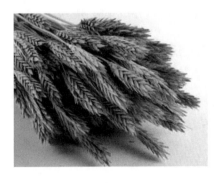

Grains are one of the primary sources of carbohydrates and include everything from bread to rice to pasta. Carbohydrates are, in turn, the primary source of fuel for the body. They are the clean burning fuel – unlike proteins which require sufficient water to wash the waste products out of your system. There are many choices in grains that are also great sources of calcium including cornmeal and several fortified cereals.

Making smart choices in the grain family, however, is probably more difficult than any other group of foods. Your local grocery store is probably stocked with thousands of products that would constitute a 'bad' grain choice because they've been made of processed white flours with a lot of additives such as sugars. Fortunately, there are a few grain products in your grocery store that would be a wise choice.

Read the package label closely. In addition to calcium content, you should check to make sure that you are purchasing whole grain foods if you want to make the best nutritional choice possible. Since the term "whole grain" is sometimes used a bit haphazardly, it might be wise to purchase the product with the highest fiber content.

It is the fiber content in the whole grains that causes them to be digested more slowly. Digesting white breads versus whole grains is sort of comparable to digesting marbles versus a whole freight train. The marbles pretty readily roll right over the boundary of your gut and into your blood stream. The freight train, on the other hand, must first be disassembled.

Since high fiber content will keep your blood sugar level more even, you will have a more steady supply of energy, feel satisfied longer, and tend to eat less. Again, it's the fiber content keeping your blood sugar even that avoids insulin spikes and feeling famished. Simple carbohydrates like white bread and the average pasta cause instability of insulin because they lack fiber. Avoiding this spiking effect by getting adequate fiber in the whole grains will allow you to maintain an even, constant level of energy and keep your metabolism working at its highest potential. You'll feel better and have more enthusiasm for your daily exercises (next section).

Whole grains, vegetables and fruits are a great source of soluble and insoluble fibers. Fiber is not absorbed or digested, but travels through the body in its original form, aiding in digestion and helping prevent constipation. 25 to 38 grams of fiber per day are recommended.

Water-soluble soybean fiber is one of the fibers that aids in calcium absorption. Getting a wide source of fibers from grains, vegetable and fruits is the wisest protection of calcium absorption as well as overall health.

Fruits and Vegetables

A government study into the dietary habits of the average American discovered that only 55% of Americans eat any vegetables or fruits *at all* on a daily basis. Not an apple, not even a baby carrot or a single stalk of celery! That's nearly as bad as our lack of calcium intake!

There's little wonder that health problems and chronic disease caused by dietary deficiencies are on the rise. Vegetables and fruits are a great source of dietary fiber and a source of low calorie carbohydrates to be used for energy. The vitamins and minerals they provide are also vital to achieving good health and to enabling proper calcium absorption.

Secrets Inside Bones, Brains & Beauty
Benefits of Eating
Fruits and Vegetables

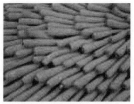

- Increases availability of important vitamins and minerals
- Promotes eye health
- **Builds better bones**
- Helps maintain good blood pressure
- Aids in digestion and overall digestive health
- Reduces cholesterol
- Helps body to utilize glucose for energy
- Provides **Phytochemicals** (plant derived substances that are the subject of intense recent research for their ability to protect against disease and prevent forms of cancer)
- Provides **Antioxidants**

The Dairy Group

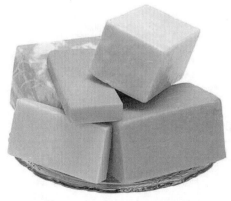

We discussed the dairy group in the last section, but it's worth repeating what a wonderful source of calcium all of these foods are. Dairy foods have gotten a bad rap in recent years. There has been an emphasis on the high content of environmental pollutants and "bad" fat. Also, lactose intolerance (with the associated sick stomach and bowels) became a more widely discussed problem.

The dairy group is currently experiencing some resurgence in popularity. Recent scientific studies have shown that getting three servings of calcium rich nonfat dairy foods a day can actually help facilitate weight loss in women who eat a sensible diet. (Hence the 'get three a day' ad campaign you may have seen on television and billboards around the nation.)

If you could possibly lose a few pounds (which many of us could afford to do) and build strong bones at the same time, there's even more reason to make sure you get an adequate intake from the dairy group.

Good Choices and Serving Sizes from the Dairy Group

1 cup low fat cottage cheese
1 ½ ounce of hard low fat cheese
2 cups of low fat processed cheese
1 cup of skim or low-fat milk
1 cup of reduced fat or nonfat yoghurt
1 ½ cup reduced fat yoghurt smoothie

Proteins

Some of the most compelling recent research regarding the connection between our diet and stronger bones is the relationship between our protein intake and our bone mineral density.

Secrets Inside Bones, Brains & Beauty
Protein can help increase bone density

When calcium intake is high enough, adding protein to the diet can increase bone mineral density. Research recently published suggests that increasing protein intake to 1.55 grams per 2.2 pounds of body weight may increase some bone growth factors. This is true whether the source of protein is animal or plant.

For example, if your weight is 150 pounds, you might benefit from 105 grams of protein per day **when your calcium intake is adequate**. Those last six words are so critical that I will restate them in the positive. **Your calcium intake must be adequate so the added protein can be helpful**.

Proteins are complex molecules. How you get them and how you use them can be a complex topic. No consensus exists on the impact of the protein you eat on your overall use of calcium and on your bone health.

However, studies have found remarkable improvements in the recovery from hip fractures in hospitalized elderly individuals who were given protein supplements. Medical complications and length of stay in rehabilitation units have been decreased. One study with individuals about 80 years old found increases in insulin-like growth factor-I (IGF-I), a marker of bone formation. The individuals in this study who were given the protein supplement lost about half as much bone mass after the fracture in comparison to the elderly who were not given the protein supplement.

Another study looked at healthy men and women over the age of 50. Again, the individuals in the high protein group (1.6 grams per 2.2 pounds of body weight per day) had significantly higher measures of insulin-like growth factor than the comparison group (0.78 grams per 2.2 pounds of body weight per day). It is noteworthy that this amount is greater than the RDA. It is also significant that the high protein group had lower measures on urine tests for bone breakdown. These researchers concluded that this increase above the RDA may have a good impact on the bones of healthy older men and women when calcium intake is adequate.

Remember that we need proteins to build healthy tissues in our bodies. This includes our bones. Proteins are necessary during building, repairing, and replacing body tissues at any age. It's no surprise that protein is critical to rebuild the structure of our bones after a fracture and to keep our immune response healthy.

Most studies looking at the spread of osteoporosis have shown a positive association between protein intake and BMD when calcium intake was high enough. One of the bad effects of a low protein diet may be related to the significant reduction in calcium being absorbed in the intestines. This makes sense because protein helps transport calcium out of the gut and into the blood.

Isoflavones are a specific kind of soy protein that may protect your bone health. The typical Asian intake is about 10 grams per day. This can be considered safe. Long term use of this source of protein has been associated with healthy bones in the elderly. As previously stated, water-soluble soy fiber aids in calcium absorption.

Protein can also be harmful to bones

By the same token, eating **too much protein** has clearly been shown to **increase the amount of calcium lost in the urine**. It has been estimated that every gram of protein intake may be associated with the loss of 1.5 mg of calcium in the urine. Thus it is important to balance the amount of protein eaten with the amount of calcium and vitamin D consumed. The recent recommendation is to increase daily protein intake to 1.55 grams per 2.2 pounds of body weight when calcium and vitamin D intake are adequate.

A positive impact on bone health is generally found in studies in which the calcium source was dairy products. This suggests no bad effect of the protein in dairy products. However, dairy foods vary widely in their content of nutrients. Some research suggests that milk and yogurt could be beneficial while cottage cheese, which has higher protein content and lower calcium content, may decrease calcium absorption.

Beyond Vitamin D Are Other Essential Vitamins

As mentioned above, fruits and vegetables are great dietary sources of many essential vitamins that are needed for good health and proper calcium absorption. Because the diets of many Americans are very low in these important foods (and because of possible nutrient loss in food due to environmental pollutants as mentioned earlier), count your intake of these nutrients closely.

You will want to make up for any inadequate dietary intake. As has been suggested by the American Medical Association's response to research, most people will need to take vitamin supplements. Through dietary and supplemental sources, make sure that you get the following vitamins.

Vitamins A, C & K

You will want to count vitamin C, vitamin K and vitamin A as beta carotene.

Getting vitamin A the natural way is considered most safe. Too much vitamin A through supplements can be harmful to your bones. Taken in the form of retinol, it may contribute to hip fractures in women with osteoporosis. However, beta carotene in higher doses did not increase the risk of hip fractures.

Vitamin C is needed to form the protein structure of your bones. Collagen is the special protein that forms the framework of your bones that minerals will harden. Vitamin C is needed to allow the collagen to create the right kind of structure. Then adequate calcium helps to harden the bones around that structure. The combination of vitamin C and calcium in adequate doses increases bone density.

It is not clear why vitamin K reduces fractures of the spine and hip in women. It does not seem to influence bone mass. However, recent studies suggest that 375 micrograms might be needed for optimal bone health. Since this is higher than the RDA, your healthcare provider can help you decide what is best for you. It's especially important to monitor this vitamin intake if you are taking anticoagulants or blood thinners. Vitamin K helps your enzymes make the structure of your bones stronger.

Recommendations for Vitamins

Beta carotene

8,400 micrograms for females & 10,800 micrograms for males

Vitamin C

75 mg for females and 90 mg for males is the RDA. However, taking more than 600 mg of Vitamin C per day has been recommended to improve the collagen essential for strong bone.

Vitamin D **(discussed in an earlier section) – base your intake on your blood levels of 25(OH)D**

The only research showing reduction in fractures combined Vitamin D with calcium supplements.
700 to 800 IU per day reduced risk of falling by 22%.
1000 IU of Vitamin D per day may be required in the elderly.
Low blood levels of 25-hydroxy vitamin D may be associated with periodontal disease regardless of BMD.
4000 IU of vitamin D per day increased wellbeing – this antidepressant effect might reduce falls.

Vitamin K (medications may influence this dose)

The RDA is 90 micrograms for women and 120 micrograms for men. However, research suggests that even 375 micrograms may be too low to prevent osteoporosis.

Section Four: Exercise to Build Better Bones

IN THE NEWS

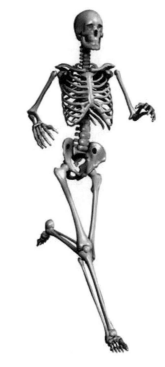

The Surgeon General's "first-ever" report on our nation's bone health includes a focus on physical activity. In <u>Bone Health and Osteoporosis</u>, the Surgeon General emphasizes the value of being physically active throughout your entire life. Done properly, this will increase the strength of your bones. It may also decrease your risk of fractures related to thin bones. As mentioned previously, go to **http://www.SurgeonGeneral.gov/** to get your copy of that report.

HEALTH TIP

Any kind of physical activity adds to your bone health. Appendix A provides a chart to guide you to some research findings on nutrition and exercise. It will list which exercises have been shown to increase bone density. Even though there are no randomized controlled studies on how exercise affects your risk for fracture, other research has found a link. These studies indicate that certain physical activities may reduce fracture risk. Even small differences in behavior can be both fun and powerful

Secrets Inside **Bones, Brains & Beauty**

in creating changes in your bone health. **Have you counted your total exercise today?**

FOCUS OF THE CHAPTER –   YES, YOU MUST EXERCISE TO BUILD BETTER BONES.

You will be learning how to move more muscles for the best benefit. The goal will be to build bone health and have fun, too.

We've become a world of sitters. This includes too many people of every age. We sit in the car or bus on the way to work or school. We sit at our desks through most of our workday. The same sitting behavior gets us home after work. And there we sit through dinner and most of the evening. Question: If I acknowledge that I'm repeating myself too much in typing the word "sit," can you explore whether you are repeating yourself too much in the behavior of putting your derriere down when you could be standing or racing around?

Regardless of your answer, I would submit to you that the best baseline measure for your activity is probably a pedometer. In fact, you might want to put this reading down until you go get one.

~ ~ ~

Did you do it?

~ ~ ~

The recent Consumer's Report evaluated several of them. Their "Best Buy" pedometer was listed as selling for $20 while their top ranking one was $35.

Certainly those would be dollars well spent. As soon as we know how many steps you take and where you take them, the sky's the limit on ideas for increasing your number of steps per day. The goal would be a gradual increase until you are taking 10,000 steps per day.

The reason for the pedometer will become more evident shortly. For the moment, let's concentrate on some of the reasons exercise plays such an important role in bone health.

Your bones are an active organ. First, they function as a warehouse. They have to do a great job storing minerals, vitamins, hormones and other things that are crucial to your ongoing health. Their other major job in your life is providing a framework of strength. This frame has to protect your softer parts such as the lungs and brain. The strength of your frame also makes it possible for you to walk safely.

The strength of your bones increases when the right demands are put upon them. In a healthy sequence, you first put just a little more physical stress on your bones than they are prepared to handle. This causes some minor damage to your bones. Science refers to this as micro-damage to the bone architecture. You follow this mechanical stress with some rest, relaxation and adequate nutrition. Your stressed bones use this rest period to repair the damage in ways that actually make them stronger than they had been. Sometimes they also get a bit bigger than they were prior to this repair of the damage caused by the mild biomechanical stress.

This is one cycle of health. All things considered, this

(minor stress -> rest and nutrition -> repair)$^\infty$

cycle done correctly and repetitively increases the bone density. It also improves your muscle strength, muscle mass and muscular endurance. This is likely to result in better coordination, the ability to move more quickly and accurately, better flexibility, better mental and physical health and improved balance.

These things may help you avoid falling. The impact of the fall may also be lessened. Please note and always remember: minor stress alternated with rest is essential.

Always. Even in youth.

People training for extreme sports or dance events can create osteoporosis simply by exercising too much. If they also eat poorly while creating too much biomechanical stress on their bones, they would be at increased risk for osteoporosis or osteopenia with low bone density and higher risk of fractures.

It is worth repeating:

**The balance of minor mechanical stress
and repair
will always be important
to your bone health.**

We know that other things also influence our bone mineral density, but adequate physical activity is essential. Yet almost nobody of any age gets enough exercise.

69

So what's the problem?

Adding physical activity on a daily basis strengthens our bones. It also can help you keep your weight in a healthy range and avoid many of the chronic diseases that used to be considered part of normal aging.

Osteoporosis is NOT part of normal aging.

Neither are heart disease, diabetes, depression and hypertension. Each of these is significantly less likely to occur in people who have been physically active on a regular basis. Each of them can also be effectively treated with a proper exercise program.

My favorite story in this realm was written in TIME Magazine several years ago. A man in his late 80s made a visit to his doctor to find out why his one knee hurt so badly. The physician said there was no need to worry. It was just the arthritis associated with aging. To that, the irate elder said, "Looka here, Doc! This other knee is also" more than 80 years young!

All things considered, a regular program of exercise may just be the best health insurance and life insurance you could ever get. And this insurance could be free! Might that be even better than putting money in the bank? Again, too few people do enough of either.

Evidence keeps coming in that life-long physical activity improves bone mineral density and decreases risk of fractures. You are never too young to begin.

Adolescence is prime time to get the most bone strength out of every exercise you do. Scientists believe that the size and structure of your bones are pretty much set during your teenage years. Your peak bone mass is created about the time you are 30 years old.

Boys tend to be more active across their lifetime. That may be part of the list of reasons why they are at less risk for osteoporosis. Boys also tend to consume more calcium during this critical growth spurt.

Unfortunately, adolescence includes so much peer pressure with regard to physical appearance that girls don't do as well on physical activity. That only accentuates their poor nutrition. Many of them go on unhealthy weight loss diets instead of an exercise program that would improve their bone health. Drinking soft drinks with junk food instead of having the milk pictured with the ginger snaps has become a national trend in the USA. This coupled with being sedentary is gradually destroying our nation's bone health. Sadly, it is also resulting in an increasing occurrence of osteoporosis globally!

One goal of this guide is to show individuals of all ages the lifestyle choices that are fun, easy, and designed to Build Better Bones. These would be choices that would serve anyone well across their entire life. In fact, it's never too early and never too late to exercise your way to bone strength for health, safety and vigorous longevity.

What choices do we have?

When you exercise, you build more muscles. Your muscle cells need more calories than your fat cells need just to exist. Mitochondria is the big word that labels the little energy factories in your muscle cells. Your mitochondria need good nutrition just to maintain what you have. As you increase your physical activity, ideal nutrition becomes even more necessary.

71

What that means to you is: If you increase your exercise while you keep your diet exactly as it has been, you will lose weight. It's the old energy in, energy out formula. In part, you will gradually burn up more of what you eat rather than storing it as fat. In addition, you will probably burn off some of the energy stored in your fat cells. However, when you improve the quality of what you eat while adding exercise to each day, you can hasten your path to overall health and healthy weight maintenance.

This is important in preventing and reversing osteoporosis because your muscle size is related to your bone density. It's the combination of eating smart while exercising right that builds bone density as well as muscle mass and muscle performance.

The bad news is described in a recent study: The percent of adults in the USA who have regular physical activity decreases with age! Can you see why this might be related to increasing medical problems with increasing age? Can you imagine how this is related to the health crisis in our nation as the "third-age" population increases in number? There's a statement that is worth repeating and memorizing:

Osteoporosis is NOT part of normal aging.

Are you duly impressed with how serious the need is to count your exercise today? 44 million people in the USA alone are at risk for osteoporosis. Most of them do not realize their risk. Most of them fail to grasp the multitude of values from exercise. Even if they get a grasp, they probably don't do it.

I remember being shocked to the depths of my soul by my friend's response some years back. When I complained strenuously about being "so tired," he said, "Maybe you should exercise." At that level of fatigue a nap was much more appealing! That was one of those moments when a friend's wisdom just didn't seem logical. Time and experience proved that advice to be true.

What is our ultimate model of hope for exercise to Build Better Bones?

The good news is that gradual increases in physical activity have been shown to improve many measures of physical and mental health. How much change is required of you? Even the Surgeon General has only recommended a "minimum of 30 minutes of physical activity of moderate intensity (such as brisk walking) on most, if not all, days of the week."

But let's get to the ultimate model of hope for preventing and treating osteoporosis based on science. Remember that it's never too early and never too late to Build Better Bones. Your age is likely to influence the amount and nature of impact your exercise program will have, but bone health can be improved with exercise at any age.

Your exercises will affect the body part you use…so walking will not make your wrists stronger. Life long exercise is essential because the effect doesn't last across an extended period of time…so you need to make exercise a regular part of your every day routine.

If you have been a couch potato for too long, the good news is that you will see more improvement faster than your athletic friends. The other news is that you would be wise to start slowly but do so immediately after your healthcare provider approves your exercise plan.

What must you do to rest assured that you are doing your very best? Put another way, what have others done to avoid or reverse osteoporosis? Appendix A can be printed as a poster to display in a prominent place so you can remember the bare minimum. Here are some of the research findings to complement those details.

Weight bearing

Women who reported standing more than 4 hours each day were less likely to have osteoporosis. Is weight bearing alone enough to strengthen your bones? Apparently not. People who are paralyzed below the waist have not shown significant increases in bone mineral density simply by standing. Adding muscle activity while standing complements the benefits of weight bearing.

Walk

Women who reported walking an hour or more a day had higher bone mineral density. Walking more than a mile per day,. or about 7.5 miles per week, was associated with greater whole body bone mineral density. You are less likely to fall if you maintain enough physical fitness to be stable and strong in tandem (heel to toe) walking. Backward tandem walking can be beneficial in measuring dynamic balance. This may be one of the ways to improve your balance after you have built sufficient strength and coordination. Having good balance would be likely to decrease your fall risk.

Typically, the research suggests that walking is most beneficial at a brisk pace. That means almost aerobic. That means your walk is rapid enough that you know you are putting in significant effort, but you are not too short of breath to carry on a conversation or hum a tune.

Weight bearing impact aerobics

Moderate to high intensity weight-bearing aerobic exercise increases bone mineral density. This is especially true with high impact. For example, jumping rope and skipping have been shown to increase bone density up to 4% in women before and after menopause.

Children have increased their bone mass and bone size with high-intensity jumping. Both the hip and spine have been affected. Jumping off an object that is about 20 inches high might be considered a safe and easy way for children to set the stage for bigger, stronger skeletons for their vigorous longevity.

How long this increase in bone density would last is unknown. Master runners have maintained for as much as 5 years. After 20 years of retirement, soccer players had lost their edge. So the examples in research are relatively clear. Start in youth. Stand at least 4 hours. Walk at least a mile a day. Jump about a bit. Use it to keep it.

Beneficial exercises to Build Better Bones include step aerobics, dancing, tai chi, hiking, stair climbing (both up and down), and activities that force your muscles to work against gravity.

Strength training

To increase your muscle mass as well as your bone density requires strength training. The recommendation is to start with weights that are relatively easy to lift. The other essential is that you gradually increase the weight of the weights you are lifting rather than the number of repetitions of lifting them.

Muscle and bone mass will only be increased at the body parts you exercise. For example, you might notice a difference in your arms because you use one more than the other. The arm you use more in day-to-day activities might show as much as 5% difference. Researchers in Finland measured arms of women who played tennis or squash. With this increased use of the playing arm, the differences were even greater. It was as high as 16%.

It is important to remember another finding of this research from Finland. Women who started training before adolescence got twice as much benefit as the women who began the sport after puberty!

Adolescence may be a time of turmoil because of the struggle for identity, peer acceptance, separation, and more. But remember, it is also a "window of opportunity" during which maximum gain can be obtained for every effort you make to achieve optimal bone health. Let the adolescents among us rejoice! They have a leg up on the rest of us for achieving the optimum in bone health. Let the frail elderly take heart. Others in their 9th decade of life have improved their bone density and decreased their risk for fractures. Let any age remember the motto: Use it to build it and keep it.

In fact, even the size of the bones can be increased in the frail elderly. Men have more advantage in this component. The biomechanical stress of increased physical activity may cause this increase in bone size. Since this strengthens the bone, this may decrease the risk for fractures in the frail elderly.

Strength training increases muscle mass as well as bone mass. While that is important at any age, it is particularly critical in aging. It gives you the energy and physical power to do what you must do in your everyday life This includes the simple things such as carrying home groceries and keeping up with the kids and grandcherubs.

It is significant that the estimated average muscle mass lost is 5% per decade after age 30 with the assumption that this may be more rapid after age 65. Current theories relate this to a variety of things.

One example is protein synthesis. It is thought that the aging body is more adept at breaking down protein than in creating it.

Another theory is that the mitochondria in your muscle cell reduce enzyme activity. As described above, the mitochondria might be thought of as little energy factories or power plants in your muscle cells.

Yet another theory has to do with your hormones. With aging you have less of the hormones needed for muscle maintenance, such as testosterone and growth hormone. Also, the decline in muscle blood flow and nerve function that come with aging may contribute.

Those are some of the theories. They tend to be based on observations of how aging has progressed in humans to date. It should be noted, however, that most of the aging populations observed have tended to become increasingly sedentary and obese in a fast food nation.

This is the good news. You can send a message to your mitochondria to increase their enzyme activity. How

77

would you do that? Increase your physical activity. Even frail nursing home residents have increased their strength and muscle performance with exercises and activities aimed at muscle strengthening.

Stretching

To move quickly and accurately enough to avoid falls you need flexibility. Stretching will help you become more flexible. This is one of the most frequently ignored parts of exercise programs. Be sure you see the value of it. Avoiding falls is critical to reducing your risk of fractures. Stretching also may reduce stiffness and soreness, increase your ability to do other physical activities and add to the pleasure in being more active.

Balance Training

Increasing muscle strength and performance may increase bone density. Improving your balance may not be associated with increasing your bone mass. However, an even more significant gain is the reduction in risk for fractures from falling. Increasing strength, improving balance, becoming more flexible, and being able to respond faster are the most important parts of your exercise program for bone health and avoiding fall-related fractures.

An exercise program that includes training in balance can reduce falls by 17%. This could translate into a huge improvement in vigorous longevity with maximum independence and quality of life.

In summary, all of the research translated for you here is provided for educational purposes only. Your healthcare provider should approve any change in your exercise program before you begin it. The more educated you are, the better equipped you will be to work effectively with your healthcare provider to design the strategy which is unique to you, your current baseline, and your goal of optimal bone health. That means the questions you ask of your health care provider will be more efficient and to the point. Therefore, your program for change is much more likely to improve your bone health.

Secrets Inside Bones, Brains & Beauty

Research shows that beneficial exercises include:

- Walking briskly an hour a day, going 7 or more miles per week

- Being physically active while standing for more than 4 hours each day

- Weight lifting with gradual increases in the weight of the weights

- Tai chi

- Yoga

- Step aerobics

- Jumping or skipping rope

- Dancing

- Hiking

- Stair climbing – both up and down

- Activities that force your muscles to work against gravity

The essential ingredients of your exercise program are:

- Consider your baseline measures when setting up your exercise program

- Remember – the less active you have been the more you have to gain by increasing your exercise activities now

- Make the most out of the "window of opportunity" afforded by youth by jumping about a bit during those years

- Continuing physical activity across your entire life

- Remember – even the frail elderly may be able to benefit by being more active

- Make exercise an essential part of every day

- Vary your exercise so all body parts increase in bone mass as well as muscle mass and performance

The main goals of your exercise program:

- **Decreased risk of fracture through long term physical activity**

- **Increased bone mineral density**

- **Increased muscle mass**

- **Greater muscle strength**

- **Improved coordination**

- **Better balance**

- **More flexibility**

- **Increased speed of reaction and movement**

- **Optimal mental, emotional and physical health**

Secrets Inside Bones, Brains & Beauty

Closing Summary and Prediction

This is the ultimate model of hope because it takes new research findings which describe how others have prevented or reversed osteoporosis and helps you learn how to apply that science to you uniquely. It empowers you to make the most out of what is known by taking **5 Easy Steps to Build Better Bones: _B O N E S_.**

- Step 1 **_B_** BASELINE measures to establish your baseline: Work with your healthcare provider to get the appropriate measures of your current level of bone health. Count your intake of all important nutrients…because you probably need to increase several of them. Determine how you currently handle stress…because you may want to become an expert in managing your mental and emotional stress. Use a pedometer and other measure of your physical activity…because you may want to increase that, too.

- Step 2 **_O_** ORGANIZE your unique winners strategy…so you CAN Build Better Bones. Your baseline measures will show you some things to celebrate…and identify what you need to change. Optimal health is not a "one size fits all" kind of situation.

- Step 3 **_N_** Now! DO it NOW! DO it with relish…so you can find new and different ways to manage stress, exercise for overall fitness, and eat for fun and bone health, too.

- Step 4 **_E_** Evaluate & REWARD. Give yourself a lot of positive reinforcement for progress…so you can stay on track. Start small and reinforce big with a lot of compliments from your own small voice within.

Secrets Inside Bones, Brains & Beauty

You're the only human being that will ever spend twenty-four hours a day with you. It is fitting and effective to compliment and thank yourself for each small step taken for optimal health. The time to begin treating yourself as well as you treat your best friend is now. Once again, remember...**osteoporosis is NOT part of normal aging.**

- Step 5 **S** START OVER again from Step 1...so measures of changes in your bone health can keep getting better by making the most of science. Remember...it's never too early and never too late to Build Better Bones.

B – Baseline measures.

O – Organize YOUR options.

N – Now. Do it NOW!

E – Evaluate AND REINFORCE PROGRESS.

S – Start again from your new baseline measures.

Bones, Brains & Beauty™

Prediction of a New Definition of Optimal Health

What follows is based on what I learned reading thousands of pages of research on osteoporosis and other so-called expected changes of "normal aging." Science brings new and valuable information constantly. We're wise to use it.

Additionally, there are the experiences of individuals like the 80+ year old man quoted above. One leg didn't hurt and the other did. The physician advised him to simply see that as normal aging. He countered with irritation: "Looka here, Doc! This other knee is also" well past 80 years young!

Also, information about how lifestyle choices are ruining the health of most Americans and multitudes of others around the globe is rapidly becoming common knowledge. Attempts to influence people to improve their health flood all of our senses. Even cereal boxes that contain the same fat-free cereal that they always sold now proclaim in big, bold letters: **"Fat Free!"**

We're encouraged to get back to the "Good Ol' Days" by moving our bodies more and eating less while still eating smart. We're told to learn from the celebrated centenarians found in small pockets in various countries. Model after them. Get back to the land and simple foods.

But there are many other factors that add up to the ultimate model of hope proposed herein. Several of these are important to your bone health.

It is encouraging that more people are living longer. Many of those are enjoying better health than would have been predicted by looking at the degenerative diseases that are debilitating and lead to an early death in their contemporaries. Some members of our population are showing the obese majority that vigorous longevity is a reality that can be enjoyed.

It is exhilarating to watch the increasing trend for scientists to ask a different kind of question. From the many studies on centenarians has come a variety of findings on how to live to be 100 years old and be glad you did. Now scientists are asking, "If this is good, what would optimal look like?"

In bone health, some have done that by increasing nutrients such as calcium, vitamin D and protein above the ordinarily recommended level. Others have done that by changing the amount or intensity of exercise. For example, having children jump off a structure that is about 20 inches high did show bigger and stronger bones in those children following their period of episodic jumping.

Another factor is the information explosion made possible by the internet. Anyone anywhere in the world who has access to a computer and the web has access to more information faster than was ever available before in the history of the human race. Much of that information is free.

Scientists at major research centers now have instant access to findings from researchers around the world! What this can do to accelerate the speed and effectiveness of developing solid research on the so-called diseases of aging is awe-inspiring. This will only improve when current research develops the new computer which will operate at the speed of light.

It's more efficient these days to raise questions about optimal health when so much information is instantly available and consultation can take place in real time. 25 years of research on the centenarians in Okinawa has already yielded a great deal of information about one style of optimal health. See *The Okinawa Program* by Willcox, Willcox & Suzuki for those details. Some of the guesswork won't be necessary.

The nuns of Mankato Minnesota have given us another very rich supply of information on healthy aging. The book <u>Aging with Grace</u> by David Snowdon is a lovely portrayal of the effect of choosing to stay active in every sense. That research clarifies some of the factors related to remaining vigorous past the age of 100…and celebrating that. Other populations of healthy elders also add to this rich database.

My prediction is that research is guiding us to a new level of optimal health that will exceed what has been recorded in any of the centenarian research. I'm predicting that "We haven't seen anything yet" in terms of what we can create with our bones, our brains, and our brawn. What's delicious about that is that beauty and general health improve with the measures recommended in the book you are reading. Those are side effects to live for!

Extensive research is even telling us what might cause your brain to create new brain cells! For example, exercise is a powerful inducer of growing new brain cells. So you can develop your exercise program for your brain growth, to reduce depression, to improve your heart health, and to Build Better Bones!

I believe expressions such as "bone loss that is normal for age" will become obsolete as science guides us to choices that enhance vigorous longevity. Then that finding of "normal for age" will fit differently for those who enjoy optimal health than it will for the sitters among us.

I believe that such findings as "5% decrease in muscle mass for each decade of life after age 30" will be modified when those who sit too much are the minority instead of the majority of our population.

I predict that increasing numbers of hardy folks will live to 120 or more, that they will enjoy a level of vigorous longevity that is a pleasure to observe and that they will celebrate a life well lived right through to the end.

But don't take my word for it.

Take your own health in your own hands. Educate yourself regularly for the joy and health of it. Personal empowerment is your ticket.

Use it.

Confer with your healthcare provider to establish your baseline and design a program tailored to your unique strengths and needs. Then follow those 5 Easy Steps to show how you can exceed your own personal best.

If you need a mentor to assist you on these new efforts, there would be a certain wisdom in getting one. Remember: The best and the greatest of successful people throughout history needed a team. Even Flossy Nightingale had helpers during the Crimean War.

Here's to your optimal health and abundant joy as you *Build Better Bones!* Feel free to email recipe suggestions, brief questions and comments to me at *DrJoyce@StressPower.com*. I encourage you to share this ultimate model of hope with your friends. Refer them to *http://www.BonesBrainsAndBeauty.com* so they can take advantage of having their own copy of this *Secrets Inside Bones, Brains & Beauty*.

Respectfully,

Dr. Joyce

Joyce Shaffer, PhD
Empowerment Expert

Bones, Brains & Beauty™

Secrets Inside Bones, Brains & Beauty

References

This is a partial list of the articles read in preparation for this writing. They can be accessed through libraries as well as online. A favorite site to access information on PubMed is **http://www.ncbi.nlm.nih.gov/**.

Barnes S (2003). "Phyto-oestrogens and osteoporosis: what is a safe dose?" *British Journal of Nutrition* 89)S1):898-906.

Bischoff-Ferrari HA, B Dawson-Hughes, WC Willett, HB Stachelin, MG Bazemore, RY Zee and JB Wong (2004). "Effect of vitamin D on falls." *Journal of the American Medical Association* 291(N16):1999-2006.

Bischoff-Ferrari, HA, WC Willett, JB Wong, E Giovannucci, T Dietrich and B Dawson-Hughes (2005). "Fracture prevention with vitamin D supplementation: A meta-analysis of randomized controlled trials." *Journal of the American Medical Association* 293(N18):2257-2264.

Blum, M, SS Harris, A Must, SM Phillips, WM Rand and B Dawson-Hughes (2002). "Household tobacco smoke exposure is negatively associated with premenopausal bone mass." *Osteoporosis International* 13:663-668.

Booth, SL, KE Broe, DR Gagnon, KL Tucker, MT Hannan, RR McLean, B Dawson-Hughes, PWF Wilson, LA Cupples and DP Kiel (2003). "Vitamin K intake and bone mineral density in women and men." *American Journal of Clinical Nutrition* 77:512-516.

Chapuy MC, R Pamphile, E Paris, C Kempf, M Schlichting, S Arnaud, P Garnero and PJ Meunier (2002). "Combined calcium and vitamin D3 supplementation in elderly women: confirmation of reversal of secondary hyperparathyroidism and hip fracture risk: The Decalyos II Study." *Osteoporosis International* 13:257-264.

Cummings SR, MC Nevitt, WS Browner, K Stone, KM Fox, KE Ensrud, J Cauley, D Black and TM Vogt (1995). "Risk factors for hip fracture in white women." *New England Journal of Medicine* 332(12):767-73.

Dargent-Molina P, F Favier, H Grandjean, C Baudoin, AM Schott, E Hausherr, PJ Meunier and G Breart for EPIDOS Group (1996). "Fall-related factors and risk of hip fracture: the EPIDOS prospective study." *Lancet* 348:145-149.

Dawson-Hughes B, SS Harris, H Rasmussen, L Song and GE Dallal (2004). "Effect of dietary protein supplements on calcium excretion in healthy older men and women." *Journal of Clinical Endocrinology & Metabolism* 89(3):1169-1173.

Dawson-Hughes B, RP Heaney, MF Holick, P Lips,, PJ Meunier and R Vieth (2005). "Estimates of optimal vitamin D status." *Osteoporosis International* 16:713-716.

Hall SL and GA Greendale (1998). "The relation of dietary vitamin C intake to bone mineral density: Results from the PEPI study." *Calcified Tissue International* 63:183-189.

Heinonen A, P Kannus, H Sievanen, P Oja, M Pasanen, M Rinne, K Uusi-Rasi and I Vuori (1996). "Randomised controlled trail of effect of high-impact exercise on selected risk factors for osteoporotic fractures." *Lancet* 348:1343-1347.

Nordin BEC, JM Wishart, PM Clifton, R McArthur, F Scopacasa, AG Need, HA Morris, PD O'Loughlin and M Horowitz (2004). "A longitudinal study of bone-related biochemical changes at the menopause." *Clinical Endocrinology* 61:123-130.

Nordin BEC, PD O'Loughlin, AG Need, M Horowitz and HA Morris (2004). "Radiocalcium absorption is reduced in postmenopausal women with vertebral and most types of peripheral fractures." *Osteoporosis International* 15:27-31.

Nordin BEC (2003). "Should the treatment of osteoporosis be more selective?" *Osteoporosis International* 14:99-102.

Pro-Risquez A, SS Harris, L Song, S Rudicci, B Barnewolt and B Dawson-Hughes (2004). "Calcium supplement and osteoporosis medication use in women and men with recent fractures." *Osteoporosis International* 15_689-694.

Rapuri PB, JC Gallagher, HK Kinyamu and KL Ryschon (2001). "Caffeine intake increases the rate of bone loss in elderly women and interacts with vitamin D receptor genotypes." *American Journal of Clinical Nutrition* 74:694-700.

Schurch M-A, R Rizzoli, D Slosman, L Vadas, P Vergnaud and J-P Bonjour (1998). "Protein supplements increase serum insulin-like growth factor-I levels and attenuate proximal femur bone loss in patients with recent hip fracture." *Annals of Internal Medicine* 128(Is10):801-809.

Sinaki M, E Itoi, HW Wahner, P Wollan, R Gelzcer, BP Mullan, DA Collins and SF Hodgson (2002). "Stronger back muscles reduce the incidence of vertebral fractures: A prospective 10 year follow-up of postmenopausal women." *Bone* 30(No6):836-841.

Snowdon, D (2001). *Aging with GRACE: What the Nun Study Teaches Us About Leading Longer, Healthier, and More Meaningful Lives*. New York: Bantam Books.

Szule P, F Munoz, F Marchand, MC Chapuy and PD Delmas (2003). "Role of vitamin D and parathyroid hormone in the regulation of bone turnover and bone mass in men: The MINOS Study." *Calcified Tissue International* 73:520-530.

US Department of Health and Human Services (2004). *Bone Health and Osteoporosis: A Report of the Surgeon General.* Rockville, MD: US Department of Health and Human Services, Office of the Surgeon General.

Vieth R, S Kimball, A Hu and PG Walfish (2004). "Randomized comparison of the effects of the vitamin D3 adequate intake versus 100 mcg (4000 IU) per day of biochemical responses and the wellbeing of patients." *Nutrition Journal* 3(1):8.

Willcox BJ, Willcox DC & Suzuki M (2001). *The Okinawa Program: How the World's Longest-Lived People Achieve Everlasting Health – And How You Can, Too.* New York: Clarkson Potter.

Appendix A:
Bone Health Guide to Nutrition and Exercise

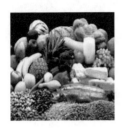
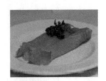
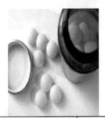

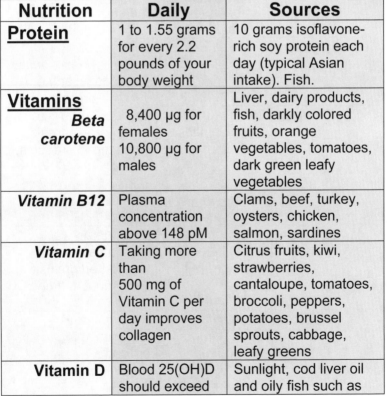

Nutrition	Daily	Sources
Protein	1 to 1.55 grams for every 2.2 pounds of your body weight	10 grams isoflavone-rich soy protein each day (typical Asian intake). Fish.
Vitamins *Beta carotene*	8,400 µg for females 10,800 µg for males	Liver, dairy products, fish, darkly colored fruits, orange vegetables, tomatoes, dark green leafy vegetables
Vitamin B12	Plasma concentration above 148 pM	Clams, beef, turkey, oysters, chicken, salmon, sardines
Vitamin C	Taking more than 500 mg of Vitamin C per day improves collagen	Citrus fruits, kiwi, strawberries, cantaloupe, tomatoes, broccoli, peppers, potatoes, brussel sprouts, cabbage, leafy greens
Vitamin D	Blood 25(OH)D should exceed	Sunlight, cod liver oil and oily fish such as

	72 nmol/L, may require up to 1000 IU a day.	salmon, mackerel and sardines 3 to 4 times a week.
Vitamin K	375 micrograms or more if indicated	Deep green vegetables, soybean oil, and some cheeses.
Minerals **Calcium**	Children 800 to 1200 mg Adolescents & young adults 1200 to 1500 mg Adults 1000 mg Adults ages 50+ 1000 to 1500 mg or more as indicated	Milk, milk products, corn tortillas, calcium-set tofu, Chinese cabbage, kale, broccoli, juices and milk fortified with Calcium Citrate Malate. Take **Calcium Citrate Malate** supplements.
Phosphorus	1,206 to 2276 mg	Milk, yogurt, ice cream, cheese, peas, meat, eggs, some cereals, breads
Copper	700 to 1300 µg Upper Limit is 10,000	Seafood, nuts, seeds, wheat bran cereals, whole grain products, cocoa
Zinc	8 mg for females & 11 mg for males	Fortified cereals, red meats, and certain seafood
Manganese	1.8 mg for females & 2.3 mg for males	Green leafy vegetables, unpolished grains, nuts, meat, starches, milk
Boron	No RDA but the Upper Limit is 20 mg	Fruit, potatoes, legumes, milk, avocado, peanut putter, peanuts

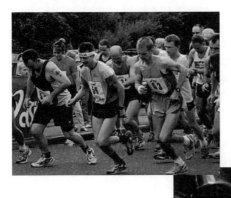

Exercise

Follow your healthcare providers' recommendations about exercise.

These research findings associated with higher BMD and lower rates of fractures are presented for educational purposes only.

WALK 1 hour a day – briskly. Wear a pedometer and build up to **10,000 steps per day**.

STAND more than 4 hours a day… add **MUSCLE ACTIVITY, too**.

Gradually increase the WEIGHT of the WEIGHTS you lift in strength training rather than the frequency of lifting them…to increase your Bone Mineral Density (BMD).

Moderate to high intensity **weight-bearing aerobic exercise**, high intensity progressive resistance training, and **high impact loading (such as jumping)** *increased Bone Mineral Density by up to 4%* in pre- and postmenopausal women.

Beneficial exercises include:

- weight-lifting

- tai chi

- step aerobics

- dancing

- hiking

- stair-climbing (up and down)

- activities that force your muscles to work against gravity.

Your exercise goals are a long term history of physical activity for:

- Increased Bone Mineral Density

- Decreased risk of fracture

- Stronger muscles with more muscle mass

- Better coordination

- Improved balance

- Greater flexibility

- Maximum agility

- Faster Reaction Time

- Balance training

Appendix B: The Bone and Joint Decade

Celebrate the Bone & Joint Decade for your bone health

The best way to address osteoporosis in man and in woman is prevention. This is increasingly critical to defuse the global osteoporosis time bomb. Prevention would be especially beneficial since many of the interventions to maximize, preserve and even improve bone health are cost effective while bringing multiple health benefits.

For example, many of these, or similar, lifestyle changes that address osteoporosis address the issues of the metabolic syndrome at the same time. For more information on this and related topics make frequent visits to **http://www.BonesBrainsAndBeauty.com** where new research will be described. Like osteoporosis, the metabolic syndrome in men and in women is having devastating consequences around the world. Specific to osteoporosis, the aim of prevention is to avoid the first and all subsequent potential fractures in safe and cost-effective ways that reduce total morbidity and mortality.

The international Bone and Joint Decade (2001–2010), endorsed by the World Health Organization, provides an opportunity to launch a strategic plan for prevention and reversal of osteoporosis. In concert with the huge and building epidemic of osteoporosis, its devastating human and economic burden, and the morbidity and mortality rates associated with osteoporotic fractures in the USA, two recommendations are made here:

Secrets Inside **Bones, Brains & Beauty**

1. Osteoporosis should be adopted by the Federal Government as a National Health Priority Area with commensurate funding. This should include funding new research, implementing policies and campaigns to increase public awareness of the need for beneficial nutritional and physical activity and developing well-structured plans to make these programs easy, enjoyable and rewarding.

2. The Federal Government should support a National Strategic Plan for urgent implementation during the international Bone and Joint Decade.

Appendix C – Some of the factors, tests and measures that might be part of establishing your baseline:

Age

Resting pulse

Height – especially loss of more than 1 inch

Weight – especially loss of more than 1% per year in the elderly

Family history of fracture

Your medical history, especially of low trauma fractures

DXA bone scan to determine bone mineral density – the "gold standard" for diagnosing osteoporosis, osteopenia and fracture risk.

Radiocalcium absorption

Blood
- Calcium
- Alkaline phosphatase
- Parathyroid hormone (PTH)
- Cortisol
- Estrogen
- Thyroid Stimulating Hormone (TSH)
- 25(OH)D, a measure of vitamin D
- Measures of bone turnover, such as hydroxyproline or n-telopeptide
- Measures of bone formation, such as IGF-1
- C-Reactive Protein, a measure of inflammation
- Interleukin 6 master chemical for inflammation
- Interleukin 10 master chemical for repair & growth

Urine
- 24-hour urine calcium for less than 300 mg per day
- 24-hour urine creatinine for muscle mass
- Fasting calcium/creatinine ratio – second voided urine specimen after sleeping and before breakfast
- Sodium/creatinine ratio – to see if calcium loss is only due to high salt intake
- Measures of bone turnover, such as hydroxyproline or n-telopeptide

Sense of wellbeing versus depression

Secrets Inside Bones, Brains & Beauty
Appendix D – Medications for Osteoporosis

Antiresorptive Therapy – medications that reduce the effectiveness of the osteoclasts such that they break down less bone.

Biphosphonates
Alendronate (Fosamax®)
Residronate (Actonel®)
Ibandronate
Etidronate (not FDA approved; available in Canada and other countries)

Hormone Therapy
Estrogen
Estrogen & Progesterone

Selective Estrogen Receptor Modulators (SERMs)
Raloxifene (Evista®) – the only FDA approved SERM
Tamoxifen

Calcitonin
This hormone is secreted by some cells in the thyroid gland. It influences the osteoclasts to break down less bone.

Anabolic Therapy – influencing the osteoblasts to build more bone.
Parathyroid hormone (PTH)

Appendix E: Adding Calcium to your Diet

Calcium-Rich Recipe Tricks to Build Better Bones

- Substitute nonfat plain yoghurt with any foods that go well with sour cream or mayonnaise.

- Add an ounce of Romano cheese or ½ cup ricotta cheese to top off pasta.

- Use nonfat milk with stevia and fresh fruit to create a frothy delight in a blender.

- Add 2 tablespoons of nonfat dry milk powder to increase calcium and protein.

- Use nonfat milk in lieu of water to cook hot cereal or soups.

- Make canned salmon, herring or sardines a frequent ingredient in sandwiches, salads and recipes.

- Use tofu or tempeh liberally.

- Include broccoli, kale, okra and turnip greens in your meals.

CALCIUM EQUIVALENTS (each equals 300 mg of calcium)

Milk	1 cup
Yoghurt (low-fat, nonfat)	1 cup
Cheese, hard	1 ½ ounces
Romano cheese	1 ounce
Ricotta cheese, part skim, regular	1/2 cup
Cottage cheese	2 cups
Powdered skim milk	1/4 cup
Frozen yogurt, milk based	1 1/2 cups
Pudding, low-fat, nonfat	1 cup
Calcium-fortified soy milk	1 3/4 cups
Calcium-fortified orange juice	1 cup
Soy beans	1 3/4 cups
Canned salmon with bones	3 ounces
Sardines with bones	6 average-sized
Tofu processed with calcium	6 ounces
Bak Choy, dandelion greens, kale, okra	2 cups

All material herein is the exclusive intellectual property of the author and may not be copied or distributed except through written permission of the author.

All photographic images are the property of the author, morguefile.com, stock exchange photography, pixel perfect photography, or J. Iglesias photography. No image may be copied, modified, or distributed outside the bounds of this book.

Violation of these terms will result in legal action.

Bones, Brains & Beauty™, LLC

Secrets Inside Bones, Brains & Beauty

About the Author:

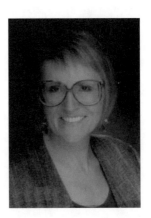

Dr Joyce is an Empowerment Expert, Psychologist, Author, Nurse & Speaker. She earned a Masters Degree in Psychology from Towson State University in 1974. She graduated from Hofstra University with a Masters and a Doctorate in Psychology in 1979. She also earned Diplomate status with the American Board of Professional Psychology.

Dr. Joyce is uniquely qualified to write and speak on osteoporosis, or "brittle, thinning bones." She has worked and conducted research in healthcare since 1961. Most of her career has been in major medical centers and universities. Since 1982 she has served in court systems as an expert on medical and psychiatric matters and had a private practice. This has kept her at the cutting-edge of research and clinical issues. Currently, she is a Clinical Associate Professor at the University of Washington in Seattle serving as a court evaluator.

Bones, Brains & Beauty™, LLC